Pharmacoeconomics in Psychiatry

Pharmacoeconomics in Psychiatry

Edited by

David Taylor MSc MRPharmS
*Chief Pharmacist, South London and Maudsley NHS Trust;
and Honorary Senior Lecturer, Institute of Psychiatry
London, UK*

Martin Knapp BA MSc PhD
*Professor of Health Economics and Director of the Centre for
the Economics of Mental Health (CEMH)
Institute of Psychiatry, King's College London; and
Professor of Social Policy at the London School of Economics
and Political Science
London, UK*

Robert Kerwin MA DSc FRCPsych
*Professor of Clinical Neuropharmacology,
Institute of Psychiatry; and
Head of Department of Clinical Pharmacology
Kings College School of Medicine and Dentistry
London, UK*

MARTIN DUNITZ

© 2002 Martin Dunitz Ltd, a member of the Taylor & Francis group

First published in the United Kingdom in 2002
by Martin Dunitz Ltd, The Livery House, 7–9 Pratt Street, London NW1 0AE

Tel: +44 (0) 20 7482 2202
Fax: +44 (0) 20 7267 0159
E-mail: info@dunitz.co.uk
Website: http://www.dunitz.co.uk

Although every effort has been made to ensure that all owners of copyright material have been acknowledged in this publication, we would be glad to acknowledge in subsequent reprints or editions any omissions brought to our attention.

Although every effort has been made to ensure that drug doses and other information are presented accurately in this publication, the ultimate responsibility rests with the prescribing physician. Neither the publishers nor the authors can be held responsible for errors or for any consequences arising from the use of information contained herein. For detailed prescribing information or instructions on the use of any product or procedure discussed herein, please consult the prescribing information or instructional material issued by the manufacturer.

A CIP record for this book is available from the British Library.

ISBN 1-85317-925-6

Distributed in the USA by:
Fulfilment Center, Taylor & Francis, 7625 Empire Drive, Florence, KY 41042, USA
Toll free Tel: +1 800 634 7064
E-mail: cserve@routledge_ny.com

Distributed in Canada by:
Taylor & Francis, 74 Rolark Drive, Scarborough, Ontario, M1R 4G2, Canada
Toll free Tel: +1 877 226 2237
E-mail: tal_fran@istar.ca

Distributed in the rest of the world by
ITPS Limited, Cheriton House, North Way, Andover, Hampshire, SP10 5BE, UK
Tel: +44 (0) 1264 332424
E-mail: reception@itps.co.uk

Composition by Wearset Ltd, Boldon, Tyne and Wear
Printed and bound in Great Britain by The Cromwell Press Ltd

Contents

About the contributors

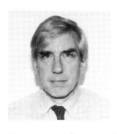

John Cookson

John Cookson won the Theodore Williams Scholarship in physiology at Oxford and obtained a doctorate in pharmacology. He trained in psychiatry at Saint Bartholomews Hopital and the Maudsley Hospital. He is a consultant psychiatrist with responsibility for an inner city catchment area, a psychiatric intensive care unit, and a specialist drug dependency unit. His main research has been in the early stages of clinical development of new drug treatments. He was a founding member of the editorial board of *Advances in Psychiatric Treatment.* With Cornelius Katona and David Taylor, he wrote *The Use of Drugs in Psychiatry* (Gaskell Press, 2001).

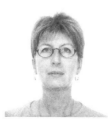

Linda Davies

Linda Davies is Reader and Director of Health Economics Research at the University of Manchester. Her research focuses on the economic evaluation of health and social care interventions in general and mental health problems in particular. Within this, specific interests include the development of methods to measure and value preferences for health and social outcomes of care, the costs of care to informal carers and the distribution of health and social well being between individuals.

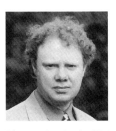

John Donoghue

John Donoghue is a pharmaceutical consultant in mental health and is a founder member both of the College of Mental Health Pharmacists in the UK, and of the College of Psychiatric and Neurologic Pharmacists in the United States. He is an honorary lecturer at the schools of pharmacy at Liverpool John Moores University and Aston University, Birmingham. His main area of research is in pharmacoepidemiology, and he is best known for a series of studies of antidepressant use in primary care in the UK during the Defeat Depression Campaign. He was a contributor to the WHO-Europe DepCare project, and has over 50 peer-reviewed publications relating to the use of medicines in psychiatry.

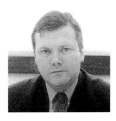

Robert Kerwin

Robert Kerwin is Professor of Clinical Neuropharmacology and Honorary Consultant Psychiatrist at the Institute of Psychiatry and Maudsley Hospital, and Head of Clinical Pharmacology and Honorary Consultant Physician at Kings College School of Medicine and Dentistry. A trained neuroreceptor pharmacologist, his main interest is the study of antipsychotic drug action using functional imaging, pharmacogenetics and post-mortem tissue. His most recent contributions have been in the elucidation of the mechanism of action of atypical drugs, development of the glutamate hypothesis of schizophrenia and the development of allelic association studies in psychopharmacology. His clinical interests are in clinical psychopharmacology and psychiatric intensive care. He is also a practising psychiatrist with a keen interest in the pragmatic aspects of drug use in clinical psychiatry.

Professor Kerwin has published very widely on many aspects on the use of drugs in mental illness. His publications include *Neurobiology and Psychiatry* (Cambridge University Press, 1995) and the *Maudsley 2001 Prescribing Guidelines* (Martin Dunitz, 2001).

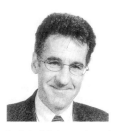

Martin Knapp

Martin Knapp is Professor of Health Economics and Director of the Centre for the Economics of Mental Health at the Institute of Psychiatry, and Professor of Social Policy at the London School of Economics and Political Science, London, UK. Much of his work focuses on the economic aspects of mental health services and health policy. He is also actively involved in work looking at economic aspects of long-term care for older people.

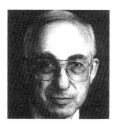

Malcolm Lader

Malcolm Lader is an external member of the Scientific Staff of the Medical Research Council, UK, and Professor of Clinical Psychopharmacology at the Institute of Psychiatry, Kings College London, University of London. Professor Lader is also an

Honorary Consultant at the Maudsley Hospital and sees patients with anxiety, sleep and depressive disorders. He is on the advisory boards of about 25 international scientific journals.

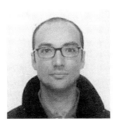

Andrea Manca

Andrea Manca is Research Fellow at the Centre for Health Economics, University of York. His research interests lie in the investigation of methodological and theoretical issues related to two broad areas: the application of modelling techniques to support the decision-making process in health care, and the use of analytical methods in the conduction of economic analysis of health care interventions. Andrea's applied work focuses on a number of different technologies in several clinical areas, including mental health.

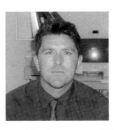

David Taylor

David Taylor is Chief Pharmacist at the South London and Maudsley NHS Trust, Honorary Senior Lecturer at the Institute of Psychiatry and Foundation President of the College of Mental Health Pharmacists. His main areas of research are pharmacokinetics and prescribing practice in mental health. His team at the Maudsley is widely involved in systemic reviews and meta-analyses of psychotropic drug therapy. David is lead author of the *Maudsley 2001 Prescribing Guidelines* (Martin Dunitz, 2001) and co-editor of *Case Studies in Psychopharmacology* (Martin Dunitz, 1998).

Preface

As the affordability of new medical technologies continues to be the subject of heated debate, so attention increasingly focuses on cost-effectiveness (the balance between costs and outcomes). Drug therapy, which is perhaps the most readily measured treatment cost, has attracted particular scrutiny.

In the case of mental illness, new drug therapies have especially been the focus of attention, partly because psychotropic medication has, for a long time, contributed little to the overall cost of treatment, but also because, with the advent of new generations of antipsychotics and antidepressants, healthcare providers are now searching for justification for the use of these much more expensive treatments.

In *Pharmacoeconomics in Psychiatry*, we have reviewed and drawn together the literature on this subject in order to explain the process of economic analyses and provide practically useful conclusions about their application to different drug groups. For this challenging task, we have enlisted the help of chapter authors widely renowned for their expertise in the clinical specialty concerned.

This book is aimed at practising clinicians, healthcare purchasers and healthcare providers. We have taken steps to make sure that the information is presented in a way that is easily absorbed and that the conclusions outlined provide the reader with helpful practical advice.

David Taylor
Martin Knapp
Robert Kerwin

Pharmacoeconomic evaluation and psychiatry

Martin Knapp

1

'Pharmacoeconomics' is a new (and not altogether elegant) word; but economic interest in drug and other treatments of health problems is much, much older. Decisions about what treatments should be available within a health-care system have always been influenced by the resources available to pay for them. Decision-makers in bygone times might not have been able to say how much a particular course of treatment was costing, and certainly would not have been familiar with incremental cost-effectiveness ratios or utility ratings, but they generally knew that they had to plan each year's spending so as to obtain the best for their patients or for the population at large.

Over time, awareness has grown of the need to secure an optimal balance (in some sense) between resources expended and results achieved. Since the late 1940s the UK has had what American observers would call a 'managed care' national health service, although not often labelled as such (Fairfield et al, 1997). Expenditure constraints and some degree of cost consciousness therefore have a long history, even if the patterns of expressed demand have fluctuated between benign neglect, hostility, blind enthusiasm and measured take-up (Knapp, 1999). Recent organizational reforms in the health system have prompted a closer look at the economics of care and treatment. For example, the introduction of the 'internal market' in the National Health Service in the 1990s made it necessary to be much more explicit about the costs and the expected effects of interventions. Even if contracts between purchasers and providers did not (initially) set prices for particular types of intervention, there was nevertheless a sufficiently major overhaul of the system of health-care funding to increase economic awareness among the main internal market 'stakeholders'. More recently, the National Service Framework for Mental Health (Department of Health, 1999) was partly underpinned by concerns about cost-effectiveness.

Over time, of course, such awareness has continued to grow, although so too has the realization that it should not be *cost* that drives macro or micro decision-making, but *cost-effectiveness*. That is, the health-care system needs to achieve a good balance between the resources it uses (the costs) and the outcomes it achieves (the effectiveness). More recent developments, such as the establishment of the National Institute for Clinical Excellence, make abundantly clear both the enduring relevance of economic considerations when deciding how to use health service resources and the pervasive need to balance economic with clinical (and related) objectives.

Economics: topic and discipline

When thinking about economics, we need to make the distinction between the topic and the discipline. There is an inherent familiarity about economics that follows from regular exposure to the topic through everyday transactions—purchases of goods and services—and through the media coverage of (for example) poverty, unemployment, government expenditure and taxation plans, and markets.

Although each of these topics is relevant when thinking about mental health services, it is (applications of) the *discipline* of economics that is the focus of this book. The discipline of economics starts with recognition of the basic problem of resource scarcity, emphasizes the need for informed choices as to how those resources are to be deployed, identifies criteria for choice from observations as to how individual people and organizations behave in principle and in practice, and suggests means by which those criteria can be both measured and achieved. Economic evaluation is essentially measurement of the success achieved by an economic system (or component parts thereof) in the pursuit of criteria for choosing between alternative allocations, or more generally in pursuit of personal and societal goals, particularly in circumstances where markets cannot be relied upon to generate efficient allocations of goods and services. Sometimes economic evaluation is referred to by more specific terms, such as cost-effectiveness or cost-benefit analysis, but strictly speaking—as we shall see later in this chapter—the terms are not interchangeable.

Needs, services and scarcity

It is not an exciting starting point: but scarcity is the root of economics, and scarcity is endemic. Who is to blame for this scarcity? Are governments not spending enough on mental health services, have health authorities or primary-care groups put too many limitations on the budgets for psychiatric treatments, or have provider trusts not given them sufficient priority? Does responsibility for scarcity lie with primary-care doctors who refer too many patients to already overstretched specialist services? Are previous cutbacks in preventive measures the real cause of today's difficulties? Is it that society is just so intolerant of mental illness that people with such disorders become marginalized when expenditure priorities are discussed? Or is the basic problem that the general public holds unrealistic expectations of what health and other services can achieve?

It would probably be possible to line up some support for each of these views, but this would risk diverting attention from the fundamental fact that scarcity will *always* be with us: that the needs and demands for interventions to tackle mental health problems will inevitably outstrip available supplies.

Criteria for choice and evaluation

Scarcity necessitates choice: how can resources be used to best effect? What criteria might we use in making those decisions? One of the most important will be *effectiveness*—the abilities of treatment and support resources to improve the health and quality of life of people with mental health problems; but, as we have seen, increasingly attention is also being paid to the costs of achieving those effects. The generic term for the criterion that combines effectiveness with resource considerations is *efficiency*. A third criterion of importance is *equity* or fairness in the distribution of access to treatment resources, the burden of financing them, or of their effects on health and quality of life.

Pharmacoeconomics needs to address all three criteria. One reason is because effectiveness, efficiency and equity are most relevant to economic evaluations; another is their intuitive appeal—we are likely to use similar criteria in spending our own personal resources; and a third consideration is that they underpin public policy in many countries, including the UK. There will often be tensions between the criteria: maximizing effectiveness may well not represent the most efficient use of resources, while efficiency and equity may often appear to pull in opposite directions. There may also be other criteria to consider: notably autonomy, liberty and diversity.

Effectiveness

Effectiveness in the sense of outcome achievement is usually defined in terms of improvements to an individual's state of health or quality of life. It can also be defined as movement towards an organization's operational or policy objectives (such as to provide services to a hundred more patients). Demands for effectiveness insights are universal: clinicians and other service professionals want to know what effects their interventions exert on symptoms, behaviour and quality of life; governments want to know what returns they are getting from their investment of taxpayers' money; pharmaceutical companies want to be able to demonstrate the beneficial effects of their products; and of course patients and their families want to know that their psychiatric problems are being alleviated. We shall see in a moment that many of these same stakeholders—clinicians, governments, pharmaceutical companies and families—are increasingly likely to be demanding proof of *efficiency* and not just effectiveness.

Effectiveness measurement is complex, for—in addition to the aim of alleviating symptoms—the objectives of most mental

health services include improvements in personal functioning, ability to obtain a paid job, interpersonal relations and quality of life generally. The difficulties of measuring effectiveness mean that many policy and practice decisions are hampered by information deficiencies. Consequently, effectiveness discussions in practice settings must often be conducted in terms of 'intermediate' and much less informative indicators of service volume, quality and patient throughput.

Efficiency

Efficiency combines the resource and effectiveness dimensions. In fact, the criterion has many different (and non-contradictory) definitions, depending on the context. For the purposes of the present discussion the pursuit of efficiency can be taken as either reducing the cost of achieving a given level of effectiveness, or improving the effectiveness achieved from a fixed budget or set of resources. Efficiency has sometimes been seen as a controversial criterion, but much of this controversy probably stems from the tendency of some policy-makers to use the term 'efficiency' when they really mean 'cheap', and to refer to 'efficiency improvements' when they really mean 'cutbacks'. Understood and employed properly, the criterion really ought to be widely accepted, particularly when used in combination with equity.

In economic evaluations the efficiency criterion underpins cost-benefit, cost-effectiveness and cost-utility analyses, although we shall see later that slightly different concepts of efficiency are being addressed in each case. Governments charged with the responsibility of making the best use of public resources are among the most ardent enthusiasts for efficiency measures, but in fact there are wide constituencies of interest and demand. For example, health service and other public sector commissioners or purchasers are similarly exercised with the task of allocating the resources under their command so as to have the greatest impact on need, which will mean weighing up the costs and the effects of deploying resources in different ways.

Equity

Equity in the use of or access to resources, or in the distribution of outcomes, can become overlooked when acute scarcity or an urgent need for (constrained) choice or rationing produces a headlong rush for what might look like better 'value for money'. Social justice was one of the founding principles of the National Health Service fifty years ago and remains an important aim today: the current UK government has put great stress on its intention to tackle social exclusion. Unfortunately, many people with long-term mental health problems find themselves on the margins of society.

The distinction can be made between horizontal and vertical equity. Horizontal equity is the equal treatment of equals: individuals with the same 'needs' should receive equivalent amounts of care or support, or individuals with the same personal means (for example, in relation to income or wealth) should bear equal burdens of funding. Vertical equity is the differential allocation of treatments or outcomes to individuals with different needs, or a differential burden of payment such as a progressive tax. Targeting services on needs is the most common example of the pursuit of greater equity, and it is therefore also legitimate to question the efficiency with which equity is pursued.

A framework for evaluation

The associations between these three criteria—effectiveness, efficiency and equity—can be appreciated using a simple framework, which also makes plain the links between these criteria and certain of the theoretical and empirical constructs widely used by economists. This *production of welfare* approach, as it is known, was developed and employed in the early 1980s in the social care context (Davies and Knapp, 1981; Knapp, 1984), but has considerable relevance for mental health discussions (Knapp, 1995). It is summarized in a simple form in Figure 1.1.

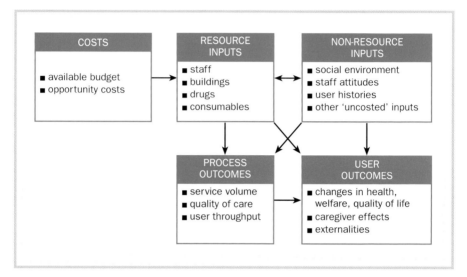

Figure 1.1
Production of welfare.

The key elements in the production of welfare framework are:

- The *resource inputs* to treatment or care: mainly professional and other staff, capital and consumables, and also pharmaceutical products.
- The *costs* of those resource inputs expressed in monetary terms or alternatively the budget for a service-providing agency which is used to purchase resource inputs, plus recognition of opportunity costs for all resources whether or not they have a price (opportunity costs are defined later).

- The *non-resource inputs* to the treatment or care process, these being the influences on the achievement of effectiveness which do not have an identifiable price because they are not marketed, and do not have an opportunity cost which can sensibly be calculated. They are not outcomes in their own right, nor are they resources to be purchased from existing budgets. Examples are biosocial influences, environmental adversity, the attitudes of the professionals delivering services, and the backgrounds and characteristics of patients.
- The *outputs* or *intermediate outcomes,*

which are the volumes of service output, almost certainly with a quality of care requirement, and perhaps weighted in some way for the characteristics of the children and young people using the service ('case mix'), produced from combinations of the resource and non-resource inputs.

- The *final outcomes*, which are changes over time in the symptoms, welfare and quality of life of patients (and their families if relevant to the context), relative to some baseline position, standard or comparator. Final outcomes are clearly measures of effectiveness. They can equivalently be defined as reductions in need.

The production of welfare approach assumes that the final outcomes of a mental health-care intervention will be influenced ('produced') by the nature of the services provided, the types, levels and mixes of resources employed, the 'social environment' of the care setting and other non-resource factors. This core theme of the production of welfare model is obviously not built up from economic theory as such, but it is a logical corollary of theory and evidence from psychology, psychiatry and certain other disciplines. However, the formalization of the links between intervention characteristics, resource inputs and patient and family outcomes owes much to economic theories of cost and production relations and their

empirical investigation. By drawing analogies of this kind it is possible to draw up testable hypotheses and to employ the empirical tools of certain branches of applied economics, including the modes of evaluation discussed in this book.

Cost-effectiveness and other evaluations
Market allocations

The simplest economic theories assume—somewhat unrealistically—that markets work sufficiently well to ensure that society's scarce resources are allocated efficiently. Of course, few markets are as well-behaved as in the elementary textbook, but nevertheless market forces can often be relied upon to allocate goods and services reasonably well between competing demands. If this is the case, then the need for economic evaluation of the costs and outcomes flowing from alternative uses of scarce resources is lessened. Mental health-care services in Britain are purchased and provided within internal markets (quasi-markets) within the state sector (mainly), and these muted market forces have clearly had some influence over allocations. Market forces have a more overt role in countries such as the USA, strongly influencing who obtains what service and at what cost to different parties. However, it is difficult to imagine circumstances in which techniques such as cost-effectiveness analysis would not be needed to guide decision-making in any of the world's health-care and related systems; that is, market forces alone are never likely to generate appropriate resource allocations or outcome achievements.

Modes of evaluation

The most commonly discussed and most useful modes of economic evaluation are cost-benefit and cost-effectiveness analyses. These and other approaches share some common elements, in particular their conceptualization and measurement of costs, but differ in two main respects: they measure outcomes differently, and consequently they address slightly different policy or practice questions.

The underlying aim of each mode of economic evaluation is to examine the efficiency with which resources are being utilized. If the evaluation is comparing two alternative treatments, the question to be addressed is whether one treatment achieves a better outcome for patients and families than the other treatment, relative to their respective costs. If the outcomes that follow from the two treatments are known or found to be identical, the economic question would be whether one treatment is less costly than the other. These are *efficiency* questions, and could be used to compare alternative accommodation settings, family support

arrangements or national policies. The various modes of economic evaluation frame these efficiency comparisons in slightly different contexts. Overlying these efficiency analyses are questions of *equity* in the availability and utilization of resources and in the attainment of health and welfare improvements. Are efficiency improvements achieved at the cost of greater inequity? Do the costs of a new policy fall disproportionately on an already disadvantaged group? Are the beneficial effects of a new treatment made available only to patients who are perhaps not seen as the greatest priorities for support?

Three evaluative modes are discussed here: *cost-benefit analysis, cost-effectiveness analysis* (and its recently distinguished variant *cost-consequences analysis*) and *cost-utility analysis.* Books by Drummond et al (1997) and Gold et al (1996)—the two most respected and widely cited texts on health economics evaluations—give excellent accounts of these modes of economic evaluation, and interested readers are referred to them for more advanced discussions.

Cost-benefit analysis

Cost-benefit analysis (CBA) is unique among economic evaluations in that it addresses the extent to which a particular course of action, such as a drug treatment or a hospital admission, is economically or socially worth while in the broadest sense. A CBA measures all costs and benefits in the same units—usually monetary units—and thus the two sides can be directly compared: if the benefits exceed the costs, the CBA evaluation would recommend undertaking the course of action; if not, it would be discouraged. The other modes of evaluation cannot provide this degree of guidance. For two or more alternative treatments or interventions, cost-benefit differences can be computed and compared: the intervention that gives the biggest excess of benefits over costs would be deemed to be the most efficient. Note, however, that the most efficient intervention may not actually be chosen: for example, equity, ideology, ethical qualms or political necessity may predominate (appropriately or otherwise).

It must be emphasized that a CBA seeks to put monetary values on one or more of the final or intermediate outcomes. It does not simply compare the amount spent with the amount saved as a result of a treatment; the latter would be a *cost-offset analysis*, which compares two different levels of expenditure. Many evaluators have carried out cost-offset analyses but erroneously given them the CBA label. Without outcome data an evaluation is certainly not worthless, but its relevance for decision-makers is generally reduced.

There are very few completed CBAs in the mental health field, and it is not hard to see why. The major difficulty is attempting to value outcomes in monetary terms.

Methodologies for this purpose have been developed by economists—for example, asking stakeholders how much they are willing to pay for different levels of a particular outcome—and are now being used in some health economics evaluations. However, there have been few attempts to explore their usefulness in mental health contexts (Healey and Chisholm, 1999; Olsen and Smith, 2001).

Cost-effectiveness and cost-consequences analyses

Cost-effectiveness analysis (CEA) is concerned with ensuring that resources allocated to the treatment of mental health problems are used to maximum effect. It is usually employed to help decision-makers choose between alternative interventions available to or aimed at specific patient groups:

- If two treatments or interventions are of equal cost, which option provides the greater benefits from a given budget?
- If two options are equally beneficial in terms of patient or population impact, which is less costly?
- If the two options have different costs and effects, what is the incremental cost-effectiveness ratio?

In the strict application of this evaluation mode, a CEA looks at a *single* effectiveness dimension and constructs a ratio of the difference in effectiveness between the two treatments divided by the difference in costs.

A generalization of CEA to multiple outcomes—which is surely necessary in an area of such symptomatic complexity as mental health—is sometimes called a *cost-consequences analysis*. In this case there is no single outcome measure to combine with costs in order to compute a cost-effectiveness ratio; instead, a set of relevant outcome indicators is weighed up less formalistically, and compared with costs. What this mode of evaluation lacks in computational simplicity (with direct implications for decision-making) it compensates for in its ability to evaluate policies and practices in a way that comes closer to everyday reality. Findings from such an analysis would need to be reviewed by decision-makers, and the different outcomes weighed up; but this is what health-care decision-makers do every day of the week, so that there should really be no hesitation among economists or other researchers about using such a technique.

Cost-utility analysis

The most recently developed mode of economic evaluation is cost-utility analysis (CUA). It is similar to CEA with the important exception that it gauges the impact of an intervention, not in terms of a single effectiveness measure such as life years gained, symptom change or relapse, but in terms of a global indicator of a patient's health-related quality of life. This indicator is labelled 'utility', and is intended to summarize more than one effectiveness dimension. Costs are measured as opportunities forgone, and represent the costs of achieving the observed changes in quality of life.

The most commonly used measure of 'utility' in the health economics literature is the quality-adjusted life year (QALY), which weights longevity by life quality. The most commonly used preference-weighted measure of health-related quality of life in the UK is the EuroQol or EQ-5D (EuroQol Group, 1990), but there are various other such measures. Utility scores can now be obtained from the 36-item Short Form (SF-36) quality-of-life scale, for example. Also in use are healthy-year equivalents (Mehrez and Gafni, 1989) and disability-adjusted life years (WHO, 2000), although both these measures are different in aim and construction from the QALY and are used less often in evaluations. It has not yet been convincingly demonstrated that QALYs *as currently measured* have validity in mental health contexts (Chisholm et al, 1997), nor that the EQ-5D or similar should replace disorder-specific quality of life measures. However, the methodological rigour and transparency of the approach is impressive, and it is certainly true that few clinical effectiveness scales currently used in psychiatric research can match the utility scales in this regard.

Cost-utility analyses avoid the potential ambiguities that can arise with multidimensional outcomes. They can also be seen as an improvement on a single effectiveness measure in what is generally regarded as an inherently multidimensional world. The transparency of the methods used to derive 'utility' is a particular strength of the approach. Cost-utility analyses are primarily justified—some would argue *solely* justified— by their use in guiding choices across a range of treatments or diagnoses: they can compare costs and impacts in two or more quite different areas of health care. This has resulted in the construction of 'league tables' of cost per QALY gained, although many people see such tables as simplistic and perhaps even capable of misleading decision-makers (Drummond et al, 1993). Thankfully, given the difficulties of justifying current utility measures in the mental health context, such tables do not extend very far into this domain. There is a danger that QALYs or similar summary measures gloss over the complexities of real-life situations. In broad evaluations CUAs are probably more useful as adjuncts to rather than replacements for cost-effectiveness or cost-consequences analyses. In the narrower setting of the decision model, some researchers have applied utility measures as a way of summarizing outcomes. Given the other difficulties that often accompany

decision models (see below), this may not be a major issue.

Putting principles into practice

The main modes of economic evaluation have a common aim in their approach to cost measurement, which—if a societal perspective is adopted (the most appropriate in mental health contexts; see below)—is to range widely across all direct and indirect costs (Table 1.1). Every resource impact and every opportunity cost are to be included. The types of evaluation differ with respect to their measurement of outcomes. In seeking to turn these economic evaluative principles into empirical studies a number of practical decisions must be taken. A fuller account of the following discussion is provided by, for example, Drummond et al (1997) and Gold et al (1996).

Design strategy

Methodologists have written whole books on research study design, and here it is possible only to touch on some of the issues they discuss. It is important to emphasize, however, that economic evaluations need sound designs just as much as any other analysis, clinical or otherwise. This is one reason why economic analyses are often supplementary to or integrated within clinical

Table 1.1
Economic evaluations: measurement of costs and outcomes.

Mode of evaluation	Cost measurement	Outcome measurement
Cost-benefit analysis	Comprehensive	Monetary valuation of outcomes
Cost-effectiveness analysis	Comprehensive	One outcome only
Cost-consequences analysis	Comprehensive	Multiple outcomes measured
Cost-utility analysis	Comprehensive	Summary utility score of outcomes
Cost-offset analysis	Comprehensive	No outcomes measured

trials. Another reason is the substantially reduced cost of completing the work.

The randomized, controlled trial (RCT) is widely regarded as the preferred design in clinical work. It is also highly desirable for economic evaluations. There are no grounds for arguing against the RCT in the mental health area, but other design strategies do also have their benefits. Naturalistic designs, whether simple before–after comparisons or statistical examinations of large retrospective data sets, have the advantage of not being conducted in what may be the unreal world of the RCT. Naturalistic evidence is most valuable when viewed alongside RCT evidence. An approach favoured by some economists in the early stages of their work is the building of decision models (Brennan and Akehurst, 2000). These are flow diagrams representing choices or routes through a care system, with outcomes and costs assigned to each end point and probabilities assigned to each of the branches (routes). In some health services research, decision models have become quite sophisticated. They are valuable for explicating the assumptions made when prospective data are not available (or not available for the full range of scenarios that the evaluator wishes to examine), but they do have their drawbacks, including susceptibility to researcher bias (Sheldon, 1996).

Patient selection

A related issue is the question of which patients to include in an evaluation. The most useful evaluation would be one that included all patients likely to use a service in the real world. However, in order to make evaluations feasible, and because of the need to achieve the informed consent of patients, many prospective clinical trials exclude certain patient groups. For example, many schizophrenia trials exclude patients with comorbid substance misuse problems. Patient exclusions always make it difficult to generalize from research evidence, but this can be an especial problem with economics studies, if excluded patients impose (or are expected to impose) costs that are out of the ordinary.

Masking

A desirable attribute of many clinical trials is for the patient, clinician and evaluator to be 'masked' (blind) to the treatment delivered. This has the advantage of reducing bias in responses and ratings. Masking is also attractive for economic evaluations, but a particular difficulty can arise. Because economic evaluations need to collect data on service utilization patterns, the very process of collection can 'unblind' the evaluator. (People having regular blood monitoring can perhaps be identified as being randomized to clozapine treatment, for instance.) Consequently, some clinical trials with health economics components have had to introduce somewhat convoluted data collection strategies in order to avoid 'unblinding' key players in the treatment or research processes.

Evaluation perspective

A well-conducted economic evaluation should normally aim to measure costs (and outcomes) comprehensively. If a decision is taken to measure less than the full range of costs, then this should be done explicitly and the possible implications noted (for example, if family or caregiver impacts are to be excluded, the evaluator should discuss the possible distortion caused by such exclusion). The evaluator needs to choose the perspective for the evaluation in consultation with the research funder and other stakeholders. One particular issue is whether the costs will look only at those falling to the health service, the public purse, or the whole economy. A broad perspective is usually more desirable (Johannesson, 1995), particularly given the potentially wide impact of many mental health problems. A narrow perspective runs the risk of missing or even exacerbating inter-agency coordination problems in the treatment and support of patients.

Cost measurement

Techniques are needed to record services used by patients, families and others affected by a mental health problem or its treatment. Techniques are also needed to calculate the associated unit costs. These are separate activities. Many instruments have been developed to collect service utilization data. The one that my own research teams employ and which has been widely used elsewhere is the Client Service Receipt Inventory (CSRI;

Beecham and Knapp, 2001). This instrument gathers data on service utilization, household circumstances relevant to a costing study, employment patterns and experiences, caregiver input, and income and benefit receipts. Johnston et al (1999) offer an excellent review of cost assessments in health-care evaluations more broadly.

The second activity is to attach unit costs to service utilization patterns and other economic impacts. The economist defines the cost of a resource as the value of the benefits forgone from not using that resource in its highest valued alternative use (the concept of 'opportunity cost'). Given that almost all resources are finite in their availability, any treatment or care activity will impose an opportunity cost, even when apparently provided or acquired free of charge (for example, the support provided by family caregivers). Economists usually base their unit cost estimates on the revealed market values of resources, with adjustments if necessary for durability and intensity of use. Beecham (1995) describes the general methodology employed for costing service inputs provided by a range of professionals and in a number of settings. Her account describes the approach employed in many mental health economics evaluations. For the UK, there is now an annual publication, *Unit Costs of Health and Social Care*, which provides updated costings for a wide range of health and social care services, together with guidelines as to how

these are to be employed for different purposes (Netten and Curtis, 2000).

Outcome measurement

In the chapters that follow a wide range of outcome dimensions are discussed, and measures presented, centred around symptoms but also looking at personal functioning, ability to work, peer and family relations, social networks and quality of life. A good economic evaluation would endeavour to incorporate such outcomes. As noted earlier, different modes of evaluation utilize different outcome data. A cost-consequences analysis would use the full range of outcome measures. A cost-effectiveness analysis (in the strict sense) would rely on one dominant outcome dimension (such as symptom reduction). A cost-utility analysis would look at a summary measure of outcomes, such as the preference-weighted, health-related quality of life measure developed from the EQ-5D or the SF36, or a disorder-specific quality of life measure. A cost-benefit analysis would convert outcomes into a monetary measure, for example using 'willingness to pay' methods. The attendant conceptual and practical difficulties of these different evaluation modes have already been discussed. There are, however, some general issues to be borne in mind.

- Changes in mental health, behaviour, welfare or quality of life sometimes take years to be achieved. Consequently, some policy and practice aims are rightly linked to influencing *lifetime* behaviour and long-term life chances. Outcome measurement would ideally take this long-term perspective too.

- For some mental health problems such as severe dementia, effectiveness might actually be achieved by slowing down a deteriorative trend or accelerating an upward trend. This makes effectiveness difficult to assess without a control or comparison group, or a set of norms, and emphasizes why naturalistic studies alone are rarely sufficient as an evidence base for clinical or policy decisions.
- Effectiveness is partly subjective (health care is what economists would call an 'experience good'), and ratings of it should be based partly on patients' and families' own experiences and views. However, patients may be poorly placed to express their views reliably because of their symptoms, or reluctant to do so because of the compulsory nature of their care or their fear of psychiatry or 'chemical coshes'. Sometimes families or caregivers, too, may not make reliable 'raters': they may not be as disinterested as one would like.
- Many interventions have 'multiple clients' (e.g. a patient and the patient's family; or a person who misuses drugs and the community offended by the criminal activity needed to fund this misuse),

raising questions as to whose effectiveness should be assessed (or what weights to attach to different perspectives), and indeed whose perspectives on that effectiveness are legitimate or relevant.

Other things being equal, the greater and the more diverse a patient's needs, the broader the range of services likely to be used and the greater the number of outcome dimensions that an evaluation might be expected to need in order to gauge their impact fully.

Outcome measurement is not discussed further in this chapter, but it should be emphasized that some distinctive contributions could be made by economics. These include the development of summary unidimensional measures (discussed in the cost-utility section earlier), and benefit valuation in monetary terms (with its attendant difficulties, even though valuation methods are breaking new ground). However, acceptable (and potentially insightful) economic evaluations can be conducted without resorting to utility or benefit measurement. Cost-effectiveness and cost-consequences approaches have a lot to offer, building on outcome measures which will be more familiar to non-economist researchers in the field. It is for this reason that cost-effectiveness and cost-consequences analyses, linked to drug trials, are the most likely to be used over the next few years.

Sample size and power

Careful thought must be given to the sample size for an evaluation. The methodologically appropriate choice of sample size should weigh up statistical power (which itself needs relevant prior information); the dangers of relying excessively on too small a sample versus the risk of introducing too much inter-service or inter-locality variability with a larger sample; the quality of the research data that can be obtained from a large number of patients; and the need for representativeness. A problem long appreciated in economic evaluations, but whose seriousness has perhaps been underestimated (Sturm et al, 1999), is that a sample size sufficient to power a clinical evaluation may be too small for an economic evaluation. This is mainly because the economic criterion variable (cost or cost-effectiveness) shows a tendency to be highly skewed. (One common source of such a skew is that a small proportion of people in a sample make high use of costly in-patient services.) This often means that a trade-off has to be made between a sample large enough for a fully powered economic evaluation, and an affordable research study. Questions also need to be asked about what constitutes a 'meaningful' cost or cost-effectiveness difference, and whether the precision (type I error) of a cost test could be lower than with an effectiveness test (O'Brien et al, 1994).

Length of research period

The potentially long-term implications of many mental health problems make it desirable that economic evaluations should endeavour to map the longer-term costs and outcomes of treatments. The challenge for a research study is to choose an appropriate length of study: too short a follow-up period will risk missing the full cost and outcome consequences of treatment, whereas too long a follow-up carries the risk that many participants will drop out of the study, and also possibly complicates the untangling of causal connections. There might also be ethical questions raised about keeping people in a trial for a long period, particularly if the economic evaluation needs a longer follow-up than the clinical evaluation. An important requirement for an economic study is to be clear about causal connections: cost and outcome consequences may be difficult to attribute to a particular intervention or event without careful research design.

Another requirement is to recognize that costs and outcomes in the more distant future might not be valued as highly as those occurring sooner. This is characteristic of most people's *rates of time preference*, and an evaluation spanning many years will usually need to discount later costs and outcomes back to a present value by an appropriate weighting procedure.

There is a third consideration to bear in

mind when looking at a health problem with potential long-term consequences. This is the problem of different time profiles for costs and outcomes: treatment costs might be borne immediately whereas the full effects of an intervention might not be observed for many years. This might create disincentives for funders. When resources are tight and performance is under close scrutiny, it can be difficult to justify expenditure today on treatments that will show no or only a modest impact for a few years. Even if there is strong evidence linking treatment expenditure today to favourable outcomes months or years later, the political or managerial imperative of demonstrating 'payback' may be too pressing to justify the allocation of sufficient resources to the area.

Conclusions

Awareness has grown in many quarters of the need for careful evaluation of the economic consequences—both short-term and long-term—of mental health problems. Despite the current real growth in funding for the National Health Service in the UK, the enormous pressures on health service resources make it wildly unrealistic to imagine that society could spend its way out of the present problems of under-resourcing and poor coordination. In countries with public health care systems, such as the UK, governments face many competing demands for tax revenue, and increases in the marginal rate of taxation are usually difficult for politicians to sell to the general public. Even when governments or health service purchasers are willing and able to spend more on mental health services, they will simultaneously be looking for ways to improve the effectiveness achieved from given levels of resources. The need for economic insights is likely to be a permanent one.

References

Beecham J (1995). Collecting and estimating costs. In Knapp MRJ, ed. *The Economic Evaluation of Mental Health Care*. Aldershot: Arena, 61–82.

Beecham JK, Knapp MRJ (2001). Costing psychiatric options. In Thornicroft G, ed. *Measuring Mental Health Needs*, 2nd edn. Oxford: Oxford University Press, 203–27. (1st edn 1992.).

Brennan A, Akehurst R (2000). Modelling in health economic evaluation: what is its place? what is its value? *Pharmacoeconomics*, **17**, 445–59.

Chisholm DH, Healey AT, Knapp MRJ (1997). QALYs and mental health care. *Soc Psychiatry Psychiatr Epidemiol* **32**, 68–75.

Davies BP, Knapp MRJ (1981). *Old People's Homes and the Production of Welfare*. London: Routledge & Kegan Paul.

Department of Health (1999). *National Service Framework for Mental Health: Modern Standards and Service Models*. London: Department of Health.

Drummond MF, Torrance G, Mason J (1993). Cost-effectiveness league tables: more harm than good? *Social Sci Med* **38**, 33–40.

Drummond MR, O'Brien B, Stoddart GL, Torrance GW (1997). *Methods for the Economic Evaluation of Health Care Programmes*, 2nd edn. Oxford: Oxford Medical Publications.

EuroQol Group (1990). EuroQol—a new facility for the measurement of health-related quality of life. *Health Policy* **16**, 199–208.

Fairfield G, Hunter DJ, Mechanic D, Rosleff F (1997). Managed care: origins, principles and evolution. *Br Med J* **314**, 1823–6.

Gold MR, Siegel JE, Russell LB, Weinstein MC, eds (1996). *Cost-Effectiveness in Health and Medicine*. New York: Oxford University Press.

Healey AT, Chisholm DH (1999). Willingness-to-pay methods in mental health care. *J Ment Health Policy Econ* **2**, 55–8.

Johannesson M (1995). A note on the depreciation of the societal perspective in economic evaluation of health care. *Health Policy* **33**, 59–66.

Johnston K, Buxton MJ, Jones DR, Fitzpatrick R (1999). Assessing the costs of healthcare technologies in clinical trials. *Health Technol Assess* **3**, 6.

Knapp MRJ (1984). *The Economics of Social Care*. London: Macmillan.

Knapp MRJ, ed. (1995). *The Economic Evaluation of Mental Health Care*. Aldershot: Ashgate.

Knapp MRJ (1999). Economic evaluation and mental health: sparse past . . . fertile future? *J Ment Health Policy Econ* **2**, 163–7.

Mehrez A, Gafni A (1989). Quality adjusted life years, utility theory, and healthy years equivalents. *Med Decision Making* **9**, 142–9.

Netten A, Curtis L (2000). *Unit Costs of Health and Social Care 1999*. Canterbury: Personal Social Services Research Unit, University of Kent.

O'Brien B, Drummond MF, Labelle RJ, Willan A (1994). In search of power and significance: issues in the design and analysis of stochastic cost-effectiveness studies in health care. *Med Care* **32**, 150–63.

Olsen JA, Smith RD (2001). Theory versus practice: a review of 'willingness-to-pay' in health and health care. *Health Econ* **10**, 39–52.

Sheldon T (1996). Problems of using modelling in the economic evaluation of health care. *Health Econ* **5**, 1–12.

Sturm R, Unützer J, Katon W (1999). Effectiveness research and implications for study design: sample size and statistical power. *Gen Hosp Psychiatry* **21**, 274–83.

WHO (2000). *World Health Report 2000—Health Systems: Improving Performance*. Geneva: WHO.

Schizophrenia

David Taylor

2

The pharmacoeconomics of schizophrenia is something of a battleground. On one side we have the manufacturers of atypical antipsychotic drugs who sponsor pharmacoeconomic evaluations of their products and find, to nobody's surprise, that their drugs are clearly cost-effective. Against them are the expert methodologists (including pharmacoeconomists) who are usually in some way funded or employed by national governments, and who dismiss virtually all studies published on this topic on the grounds that they are irredeemably flawed (see Robert and Kennedy, 1997).

Of course, both sides have conflicts of interest. The pharmaceutical manufacturers are keen to demonstrate cost-effectiveness, so that their relatively expensive products can be more widely prescribed. Expert methodologists, having established themselves as protectors of public interest, are perhaps equally enthusiastic in their efforts to limit prescribing costs by establishing atypical antipsychotic drugs as economically unproven. This view, in turn, is supported by pharmacoeconomic purists, who note, probably with good reason, the parlous state of pharmacoeconomic research in schizophrenia. Against this view are the opinions of many clinicians who, having observed the benefits of atypicals in practice, consider it unacceptable to continue to prescribe typical antipsychotic medication.

The controversy continues, with no clear resolution in sight. Meanwhile, more and more governments move towards policies that insist upon the demonstration of cost-effectiveness as a prerequisite for approval for reimbursement (Maynard and Bloor, 1998). This chapter systematically examines the available data in this area and, by stratifying studies according to their validity, attempts to draw clear conclusions from the most cogent data uncovered.

The data

The validity of pharmacoeconomic data is invariably diminished by two important factors: a failure to account for all direct and indirect cost outcomes, and the difficulty of assigning costs to human experiences. In schizophrenia, validity is further reduced by the near-impossibility of conducting trials over several years, or even decades, so as to approach the reality of what is usually a lifelong illness. Given these observations, it would be imprudent to act on the minutiae of data generated in even the best-conducted trials, but it may well be appropriate to draw broad conclusions.

Trial validity is also grossly affected by the type of trial carried out. In schizophrenia there are several: health-care decision models, retrospective mirror-image analyses (with or without contemporary control) and randomized, controlled trials. None of these is wholly satisfactory. Health-care decision models usually include no real patients and make many assumptions about outcome, often based on flawed data or mere conjecture. Mirror-image analyses compare cost and health outcomes before and after the use of a particular drug but are readily influenced by many factors completely divorced from those related to the effect of drugs. Without the inclusion of a contemporary control group undergoing all conditions except a switch to an atypical agent, none of these factors can be discounted. Indeed, trials with contemporary controls usually show a reduction in health-care expenditure after admission and switch to any antipsychotic drug. Randomized, controlled trials have the most scientific validity, but such trials are blighted by patient attrition and by the exposure of subjects to supranormal care and evaluation.

Health-care decision models and uncontrolled mirror-image studies provide little in the way of meaningful results to inform clinicians and healthcare managers. This chapter focuses instead on the results of the more robust controlled mirror-image studies and prospective randomized, controlled trials.

Clozapine versus typical antipsychotic agents

Clozapine is the most widely investigated of the atypicals, probably by virtue of its relatively early introduction and perhaps its unique efficacy. This drug has been subjected to all levels of evaluation, all of which have provided a more or less uniform view of its use: clozapine appears to be broadly cost-effective because its effect on bed-stay more than outweighs the increased cost of its purchase. This impression holds true for different countries and health systems (although most research is from the USA) and for different time periods.

As already outlined, health-care decision models hold little water in the sophisticated environment of evidence-based medicine. Nevertheless, two UK evaluations (Davies and Drummond, 1993; Matheson et al, 1994) do give some insight into the outcomes of using clozapine in the UK National Health Service, although model data were largely derived from the USA.

The several mirror-image studies of clozapine, however, give a rather more cogent view of clozapine's cost-effectiveness. All but one of the uncontrolled mirror-image evaluations of clozapine (Table 2.1) suggest that use of the drug provides overall savings in health-care costs, mainly through reductions in hospital stay. Only Jonsson and Wålinder (1995) suggested that clozapine increased overall costs, and this was found in a small study of only 21 subjects.

Controlled mirror-image studies of clozapine (Table 2.2) show primarily that all interventions evaluated seem to reduce health-care costs by reducing hospitalization, but that the effect of clozapine is greater. These results are more compelling than those from the uncontrolled studies, not only because of the inclusion of a contemporary control, but also because these studies tended to be larger and longer.

Despite the uniformity of the above findings, they remain less than conclusive because of the absence of randomization and masking, which allows the possibility of selection and assessment bias. There have been only two randomized, controlled trials of clozapine.

In Connecticut in the USA, Essock and co-workers randomized 227 patients to treatment with clozapine or to 'usual care' and observed treatment outcome for 24 months (Essock et al, 1996). At the end of this period 88 (64%) of the original clozapine group ($n = 138$) were still taking clozapine. All randomized participants were in-patients who were resistant to or intolerant of conventional neuroleptics. The authors presented only brief results. Discharge rates for the two treatment groups were similar, but stark differences were observed in readmission rates: 3% of patients taking clozapine were readmitted within 6 months of discharge, compared with 29% of

Table 2.1
Clozapine versus typical antipsychotic drugs: uncontrolled mirror-image studies.

Reference	Location	n	Mirror-image period (mo)	Outcome
Frankenburg et al (1992)	USA	75	6/30	Hospital stay and admissions reduced
Reid et al (1994)	USA	172	12/30	Hospital stay reduced. Savings calculated
Meltzer et al (1995)	USA	96	24/24	Hospital stay reduced. Savings calculated
Jonsson and Wålinder (1995)	Sweden	21	18/18	Symptoms improved but overall costs slightly increased
Gury et al (1996)	France	14	12/12	Quality of life improved; global costs slightly reduced
Geronimi-Ferret et al (1997)	France	37	12/24	Symptoms improved but hospital stay reduced
Aitchison and Kerwin (1997)	UK	26	36/36	Symptoms improved; global costs decreased through reduced hospital stay
Ghaemi et al (1998)	USA	20	12/12	Hospital stay reduced, savings calculated
Drew et al (1999)	Australia	37	24/36	Hospital stay and number of admissions reduced. Global costs remained the same
Percudani et al (1999)	Italy	15	12/12	Hospital stay reduced. Savings calculated

those receiving usual care. Costs were not assigned.

The second randomized, controlled trial (Rosenheck et al, 1997) was a complex study organized again by workers in Connecticut, but this time including patients from Veterans Affairs medical centres around the USA. In all, 423 treatment-refractory patients were randomized to receive either clozapine or haloperidol and were followed up for

12 months. Assessment of outcome was complicated by the inclusion in analyses of participants who stopped taking one treatment and began on another (40% of the clozapine group and 22% of the haloperidol group). Overall, patients originally assigned to clozapine had less severe symptoms, fewer severe adverse effects and fewer days spent in hospital (Table 2.3). Costs were slightly lower for those assigned to clozapine.

These two trials provide firm evidence of clozapine's cost-effectiveness in severely ill, hospitalized patients with resistant schizophrenia. The earlier study (Essock et al, 1996) strongly suggested reduced rates of readmission for patients on clozapine, but failed to examine carefully costs associated with treatments and outcomes. In contrast, Rosenheck and colleagues did take into account a wide range of direct and indirect costs, and demonstrated improved outcome with clozapine at slightly lower costs (Rosenheck et al, 1997). This advantage was evident despite the inclusion in the analyses of patients who switched treatments. On average, those switching from clozapine to haloperidol experienced worsening of symptoms and those switching from haloperidol to clozapine improved. Thus, the inclusion of these subjects in analyses is likely to have underestimated the advantages seen in practice.

When results of all types of trial data are taken together, it can properly be said that clozapine is probably more cost-effective than typical antipsychotic drugs in the treatment of resistant schizophrenia. This conclusion is in accord with those of other reviewers (Fitton and Benfield, 1993; Morris et al, 1998; Revicki, 1999).

Risperidone versus typical antipsychotics

Like clozapine, risperidone has been subjected to all levels of pharmacoeconomic evaluation. For example, two health-care models have predicted substantial savings resulting from the use of risperidone (Keks, 1997; Davies et al, 1998).

Uncontrolled mirror-image studies (Table 2.4) largely support these findings. Of seven published studies, five suggested that the use of risperidone reduced hospital bed-stay and some calculated savings in health-care expenditure resulting from this. Conversely, Viale et al (1997) calculated that in-patient savings were offset by increases in community services costs, and Hammond et al (1999) estimated a substantial overall cost increase for community patients switched to risperidone for at least 3 months.

Controlled trials comparing risperidone with typical drugs have provided inconclusive results overall. Of five non-randomized studies (Table 2.5) only one (Malla, 1998) indicated that risperidone use might result in lower costs by reducing time spent in hospital,

Table 2.2
Clozapine versus typical antipsychotic drugs: mirror-image studies with contemporary control.

Reference	Location	Clozapine/ comparator (n/n)	Mirror-image duration (mo)	Outcome clozapine	Outcome comparator	Overall outcome
Revicki et al (1990)	USA	133/51	12/24	Large reduction in hospital stay/costs	Reduction in hospital stay/costs	Clozapine ≫ 'conventional neuroleptics'
Honigfeld and Patin (1990)	USA	86/?	60/24	Large reduction in admissions and hospital stay/costs	Reduction in admissions and hospital stay/costs	Clozapine ≫ 'conventional therapies'
Pollack et al (1998)	USA	81/81	Variable	Admissions reduced by around 75%	Admissions reduced by around 40%	Clozapine > 'conventional antipsychotics'
Reid and Mason (1998); also see Reid (1999)	USA	383/233	24/up to 54	Large reduction in admissions and hospital stay	Reduction in admissions and hospital stay	Clozapine > 'traditional antipsychotics'
Rosenheck et al (1997)	USA	423	12/12	Large reduction in admissions and hospital stay	Reduction in admissions and hospital stay	Clozapine > haloperidol

Table 2.3
Clozapine: randomized, controlled trials versus typical antipsychotic drugs.

Reference	Location	Clozapine/ comparator (n/n)	Duration (mo)	Outcomes	Comments
Essock et al (1996)	USA	138/89	24	Discharge rates per year reported as: 27% clozapine 30% usual care Readmission rates: 3% clozapine 29% usual care	87 of 138 clozapine subjects completed 24 mo treatment Cost impact not accurately evaluated
Rosenheck et al (1997)	USA	205/218	12	Days in hospital: clozapine 144 haloperidol 168 Cost: clozapine $62 100 haloperidol $65 000	117 of 205 clozapine subjects completed 12 mo treatment 61 of 218 haloperidol subjects completed 12 mo treatment Total costs to society calculated

Table 2.4
Risperidone versus typical antipsychotic drugs: uncontrolled mirror-image studies.

Reference	Location	n	Mirror-image period (mo)	Outcome
Addington et al (1993)	Canada	74	12/12	Hospital stay reduced
Guest et al (1996)	Sweden/UK	31	12/24	Hospital stay reduced
Albright et al (1996)	Canada	146	Mean 10/10	Admissions and hospital stay reduced. Savings calculated
Viale et al (1997)	USA	139	Mean 14/14	Hospital stay reduced; community costs increased. Overall costs similar
Finley et al (1998)	USA	66	24/24	Hospital stay reduced. Savings calculated
Carter et al (1998)	USA	61	32	Hospital stay reduced. Savings calculated.
Hammond et al (1999)	USA	31	At least 3/3	Overall costs increased (community patients)

(interestingly, this was one of very few studies conducted in first-episode schizophrenia). Three trials suggested that costs resulting from risperidone or typical use were similar (Moore et al, 1998; Nightengale et al, 1998; Schiller et al, 1999) and one (Coley et al, 1999) found that costs associated with risperidone were double that for two typical drugs (mainly by virtue of high readmission rates with risperidone).

Only two randomized, controlled trials have been completed, and neither provides anything like compelling data (Table 2.6). Chouinard and Albright (1997) conducted a unique evaluation of a subset of patients from a previously conducted clinical trial. Subjects were categorized and profiled at baseline and end point according to clinical severity, and a group of psychiatric nurses were asked to rate various aspects of likely outcome and quality of life to each profile (mild, moderate or severe symptoms). 'Health state utilities' were then calculated: risperidone was found to provide more than double the number of quality-adjusted life years compared with haloperidol. Csernansky and Okamoto (1999) conducted a rather more conventional trial, but included no economic analyses. However, they did find that the use of risperidone substantially reduced relapse rates compared with haloperidol—an outcome likely to have a positive impact on cost-effectiveness.

Both of these studies are flawed. Chouinard and Albright (1997) conducted a trial so complex and novel that it is impossible

to interpret its findings with any confidence, whereas the second randomized evaluation produced scarcely any data of economic significance.

Overall, studies comparing risperidone and typical antipsychotic drugs are equivocal. There is a strong suggestion that risperidone is cost-neutral compared with older drugs (increased drug costs offset by lower use of hospital facilities), but this (despite being the most frequent finding) is not a consistent outcome. Perhaps supporting this broad contention is the observation that studies suggesting cost reduction with risperidone are offset by those suggesting cost increase. Clearly, data are inconclusive, and better conducted, controlled trials are definitely required.

Olanzapine

Pharmacoeconomic evaluations of olanzapine are dominated by data generated from a single company-sponsored clinical trial (Tollefson et al, 1997) and its follow-up. The large number of participants in the trial and its international nature have afforded the opportunity for separate analyses according to country or continent. Whether or not this is a valid approach is debatable.

Five health-care models evaluating olanzapine and haloperidol have been published. All five appear to have used the trial of Tollefson et al (1997) as the basis for

Table 2.5
Controlled trials of risperidone versus typical antipsychotic drugs.

Reference	Study design	n	Duration (mo)
Malla (1998)	Retrospective, naturalistic	102	At least 12
Moore et al (1998)	Prospective, naturalistic	118	At least 24
Coley et al (1999)	Retrospective, naturalistic	202	12
Nightengale et al (1998)	Controlled, mirror-image	150	At least 12/12
Schiller et al (1999)	Controlled, mirror-image	112	12/12

Risperidone details	Comparator details	Outcome
21 patients received risperidone from first episode 30 patients switched from typical drugs	51 patients received typical drug from first episode.	Subjects receiving risperidone from first episode spent considerably less time in hospital than other groups; service use lower in risperidone group and in those switched to risperidone.
75 patients received risperidone (in separate study); mean dose 5.6 mg/d	43 patients received either haloperidol or fluphenazine depot	Risk of rehospitalization: 21% fluphenazine depot 36% haloperidol depot 17% risperidone Costs similar for fluphenazine depot and risperidone but higher for haloperidol
81 patients received risperidone	78 patients received perphenazine 43 patients received haloperidol	Readmission rates: 26% perphenazine 35% haloperidol 41% risperidone Costs for risperidone double those for other drugs
88 patients received risperidone	62 patients received typical antipsychotic drug	Total monthly costs were similar: risperidone drug costs were higher, but were offset by lower in-patient costs
56 patients received risperidone	86 patients received typical drug	Total costs not significantly different; trend towards higher costs with risperidone. No difference in clinical effectiveness

Table 2.6
Risperidone: randomized, controlled trials versus typical antipsychotic drugs.

Reference	Location	Risperidone/ comparator (n/n)	Duration	Outcomes	Comments
Chouinard and Albright (1997)	Canada	22/21 (22 placebo)	8 weeks	Risperidone subjects to gain more than twice as many QALYs haloperidol subjects. Cost-utility ratio Can$24 250/ QALY	Retrospective analysis and utility estimates of randomized clinical trial Haloperidol dose 20 mg/d
Csernansky and Okamoto (1999)	USA	177/188	At least 1 year	Relapse at 1 year: risperidone 23.2% haloperidol 34.6% (p = 0.009)	No economic analysis provided

QALY, quality-adjusted life year.

predicting outcomes. Two of the models relate to UK conditions (Almond et al, 1999; Almond and O'Donnell, 2000) and present remarkably similar results. One of the models applies specifically to the USA (Palmer et al, 1998), one to Spain (Sacristán et al, 1997) and one to Germany (Spannheimer and Clouth, 1999). All five analyses suggest that olanzapine is more effective than haloperidol, while being cost-neutral or cost-saving.

Only two mirror-image evaluations of olanzapine have been published. In one study (Weiss and McCollum, 1998), 25 patients taking olanzapine for at least 6 months had costs compared for the 6 months before and after initiation of olanzapine therapy. Increased pharmacy costs were more than offset by large savings associated with hospitalization—overall cost per patient fell from US$17 900 to US$9600. In the second study (Sacristán et al, 1998) costs relating to treatment were again compared for 6 months before and after starting olanzapine, but this time the subjects were treatment-resistant. After 6 months, 12 of the 25 subjects (48%) had met criteria for response, and overall costs had declined numerically, but not statistically. Thus, olanzapine was clinically effective without engendering an increase in health-care costs.

Of several randomized, controlled pharmacoeconomic evaluations of olanzapine, all rely on data generated by the large clinical study of Tollefson et al (1997) (Table 2.7).

Interpretation of these data is made difficult by the varied sub-analyses produced and by the multiplicity of (often very similar) publications. Given the shared basis for these evaluations, a somewhat uniform outcome should be expected.

Each of the analyses reported outcomes for patients responding to and continuing treatment after the original 6-week clinical trial; that is, after the exclusion of patients withdrawing from the original trial for whatever reason (e.g. poor tolerability, lack of response). This probably introduced bias in favour of haloperidol, since there were significantly more responders to olanzapine. In the main, economic analysis was rudimentary and only hospital costs were included, although some reports also noted work status (but without calculating costs of productivity) and in one (Hamilton et al, 1999) a wide range of costs were considered. All sub-analyses suggested that olanzapine significantly reduced time spent in hospital, and some calculated small overall savings. Where measured, work status also improved significantly more with olanzapine than with haloperidol.

Overall, taking into account all economic comparisons of olanzapine and conventional drugs, olanzapine appears to be at least cost-neutral and may be cost-saving. However, the uniformity of results reported probably owes more to the reliance on a single source of data than to the reproducibility of economic

Table 2.7
Olanzapine versus haloperidol: analyses of data generated by Tollefson et al (1997).

Reference	n	Subgroup details	Duration (weeks)
Grainger et al (1998a)	1996 (933 in continuation phase after 6 wk)	All subjects	Up to 84
Tunis et al (1998)	1155	English-speaking countries	52
Hamilton et al (1999) Also Hamilton et al (1998); Edgell et al (1998)	817 (344 in continuation phase 6–52 wk)	USA subjects	52
Edgell et al (1999)	798 (400 in continuation phase 6–52 wk)	European subjects	52
Le Pen et al (1999)	275	French subjects	52

FF, French francs.

Outcome	Comments
Days in hospital 14/yr lower in those taking olanzapine	*All subjects entering extension were treatment responders*
Work status significantly more improved in olanzapine group	
Quality of life measures improved for olanzapine subjects	*Few details (conference poster)*
Suggestion of improvement in hospital expenditure but data not analysed by treatment	
Quality of life changes similar	*All subjects entering extension were treatment responders*
Overall cost saving US$388 for olanzapine (p = 0.033) generated by reduced in-patient costs	*Health-care costs only*
Clinical outcome, work status, quality of life and time to re-hospitalization all better in olanzapine subjects	*Conference poster*
Direct health-care costs significantly (p = 0.033) lower for olanzapine subjects	*Health-care costs only. Published in French*
Average cost saving FF137 per day	

outcome. The trials described here do not indicate unequivocally that the use of olanzapine is cost-effective, but they do suggest that time spent in hospital may be reduced in responders to olanzapine and that work status may improve. Further studies are undoubtedly required to establish more precisely the wider economic impact of prescribing olanzapine.

Quetiapine

There is little evidence relating to the pharmacoeconomic aspects of the use of quetiapine. In the UK, a retrospective audit of 20 patients (Lee et al, 1998), published only as a conference abstract, tentatively suggested decreased costs for those patients, largely through a reduction in hospital stay and resource use. Quetiapine may also improve quality of life (Hellewell et al, 1999). A large, randomized, controlled pharmacoeconomic evaluation is apparently under way (Drummond et al, 1998) and results are awaited.

Amisulpride

Economic data relating to amisulpride are very few, despite the longstanding availability of this drug in France. There appears to be only one published economic evaluation—a comparison with haloperidol (Souêtre et al, 1992). In this French study, direct medical costs were retrospectively compared for each drug over 6 months ($n = 160$). The use of amisulpride resulted in fewer days spent in hospital (93 days versus 106 days) and a significant reduction in direct health-care costs. Clearly, more studies are required to establish the cost-effectiveness of this drug.

Zotepine

Zotepine has been used in Japan and Germany for many years, but has only recently been marketed in the UK. Zotepine is referred to in two pharmacoeconomic publications (Byrom et al, 1998a, b), but no relevant data are provided. Two evaluations are apparently awaiting publication (Knoll, personal communication, 2001): one a 6-month comparison of zotepine and one a health-care model of outcomes associated with the use of zotepine and haloperidol.

'Head-to-head' comparisons of atypical antipsychotic drugs

Health-care decision-makers may be required not only to make economic choices between conventional and atypical drugs, but also between individual atypical agents. There are few direct comparisons of atypical drugs. This is probably a result of the marketing aims of pharmaceutical manufacturers: each has sought to establish the cost-effectiveness of their product compared with conventional drugs before looking to do battle with their closer competitors.

Direct comparisons of atypical drugs are outlined in Table 2.8. Overall, little can be gleaned from these studies. Comparisons of risperidone and olanzapine are dominated by data gathered from a manufacturer-sponsored, 6-month clinical comparison (Tran et al, 1997) applied to different settings or used in health-care models. Although olanzapine was suggested to be more cost-effective in these analyses, it cannot be assumed to be so given the shortcomings of the original trial. In particular, the mean dose of risperidone used (7.2 mg per day) is well known to cause more frequent and severe adverse effects than lower, equally effective doses. Interestingly, a comparison with somewhat restricted analysis sponsored by the manufacturers of risperidone (used at a mean dose of 3.75 mg per day) suggested that risperidone might be more effective than olanzapine (Procyshyn and Zerjav, 1998). Results of trials comparing clozapine with other atypicals are variable and somewhat contradictory. Even taken together, the trials comparing individual atypical agents offer little or no insight into relative cost-effectiveness.

Conclusion

Considerable funds, time and effort have been expended on pharmacoeconomic evaluation of atypical antipsychotic drugs and many journal articles and conference posters have been produced. Sadly, despite the quantity of work completed, little can be confidently concluded. Clozapine is probably cost-effective in refractory schizophrenia compared with conventional drugs since it seems uniformly to reduce time spent in hospital, and the resultant savings seem at least to offset increased drug or out-patient costs. Risperidone may also have advantages in this respect, but the data are less uniform than with clozapine and completed trials are less scientifically robust. Overall, risperidone appears to be cost-neutral compared with typical drugs, although reliance on flawed study designs makes it impossible to be certain about this. With olanzapine, although there appears to be a multitude of data supporting its cost-effectiveness, this is something of an illusion created by multiple publication of the same data. At best, trials of olanzapine suggest it may reduce time spent in hospital and improve work status. Data relating to other atypicals are equivocal, as are the results of trials comparing individual atypicals with one another.

At the beginning of this chapter the antagonism between expert methodologists, pharmacoeconomic purists and clinical pragmatists was mentioned. Given the inability to draw conclusive inferences from the data presented here, it would seem that the purists have at least partly been proved correct.

Table 2.8
Direct comparisons of atypical antipsychotic drugs.

Reference	Study design (location)	Drugs compared (n)
Ginsberg et al (1998)	Health-care model (Israel)	Clozapine and risperidone
Palmer et al (1998)	Health-care model based on Tran et al (1997) (USA)	Olanzapine and risperidone
Wieselgren et al (1999)	Health-care model based on Tran et al (1997) (applied to Swedish systems)	Olanzapine and risperidone
Spannheimer et al (1999)	Health-care model based on Tran et al (1997) (applied to German systems)	Olanzapine and risperidone
Procyshyn and Zerjav (1998)	Retrospective chart review (Canada)	Olanzapine (30) and risperidone (30)
Thompson (1996)	Mirror image— 1 yr/1 yr (USA)	Clozapine (20) and risperidone (20)
Del Paggio and Douglas (1998)	Mirror image— 6 mo/6 mo (USA)	Olanzapine (46) and risperidone (28)
Conley et al (1999)	Prospective, naturalistic—2 yr (USA)	Clozapine (49) and risperidone (75)
Grainger et al (1998b)	Data from randomized, controlled trial of Tran et al (1997) (USA)	Olanzapine and risperidone (339 in total)
Gregor et al (1999)	Randomized, controlled trial, similar to Tran et al (1997) (Australia and New Zealand)	Olanzapine (32) and risperidone (33)

Outcome	Comments
Complex outcomes dependent on assumptions made	In Israel, purchase cost of risperidone is higher than for clozapine
Analyses favour use of clozapine	
Olanzapine suggested to be more cost-effective —costs were lower and relapses fewer	Five-year predictions based on 6-mo trial
As above	As above
As above	As above
Brief economic analyses suggested risperidone associated with lower acquisition costs, but significantly better efficacy	Response rate markedly higher for risperidone (60% vs 26.7%)
Costs 3 times higher with clozapine than with risperidone	Subjects with refractory schizophrenia
Costs halved with risperidone, but doubled in those switched to clozapine	Abstract only
Olanzapine use resulted in substantial decrease in overall costs; risperidone gave rise to an increase of similar magnitude	Obscure journal source
Readmission rates at 2 yr: clozapine 13% risperidone 34%	No economic analysis
No significant differences in health-care resource expenditure	
No significant differences in health-care resource expenditure	Subjects may have been included in original trial of Tran et al (1997)

Search details

A search of Medline, EMBASE and PsycLIT was conducted in August 2000, using the following terms: Amisulpride, clozapine, olanzapine, risperidone, sertindole, zotepine, ziprasidone, economics, healthcare, costs. All manufacturers of atypical antipsychotic drugs were contacted in April 2000 and asked to supply primary reference data on their product, and all companies had complied with this request by August 2000. A further manual search was conducted of files and journals kept in the National Centre for Information on Psychotropics at the Maudsley Hospital. Reference sections from all retrieved papers were scrutinized for further relevant references.

References

Addington DE, Jones B, Bloom D, et al (1993). Reduction of hospital days in chronic schizophrenic patients treated with risperidone: a retrospective study. *Clin Ther* 15, 917–26.

Aitchison KJ, Kerwin RW (1997). Cost-effectiveness of clozapine: a UK clinic-based study. *Br J Psychiatry* 171, 125–30.

Albright PS, Livingstone S, Keegan DL (1996). Reduction of healthcare resource utilisation and costs following the use of risperidone for patients with schizophrenia previously treated with standard antipsychotic therapy: a retrospective analysis using the Saskatchewan Health Linkable Databases. *Clin Drug Invest* 11, 289–99.

Almond S, O'Donnell O (2000). Cost analysis of the treatment of schizophrenia in the UK: a comparison of olanzapine and haloperidol. *Pharmacoeconomics* 17, 383–9.

Almond S, O'Donnell O, McKendrick J (1999). A cost analysis of olanzapine compared with haloperidol and risperidone in the treatment of schizophrenia in the UK. Poster presented at the 12th Congress of the European College of Neuropsychopharmacology, London, 21–25 September 1999.

Byrom WD, Kilpatrick AT, Garratt CJ (1998a). The perceived costs of newer antipsychotics may be unfounded – Predictions of a decision-free model. Poster presented at 11th ECNP Congress, Paris, 31 October–4 November 1998.

Byrom WD, Garratt CJ, Kilpatrick AT (1998b). Influence of antipsychotic profile on cost of treatment of schizophrenia: a decision analysis approach. *Intl J Psychiatry Clin Prac.*

Carter C, Stevens M, Durkin M (1998). Effects of risperidone therapy on the use of mental health care resources in Salt Lake County, Utah. *Clin Ther* 20, 352–63.

Chouinard G, Albright PS (1997). Economic and health state utility determinations for schizophrenic patients treated with risperidone or haloperidol. *J Clin Psychopharmacol* 17, 298–307.

Coley KC, Carter CS, DaPos SV, et al (1999). Effectiveness of antipsychotic therapy in a naturalistic setting: a comparison between risperidone, perphenazine, and haloperidol. *J Clin Psychiatry* 60, 850–6.

Conley RR, Love RC, Kelly DL, et al (1999). Rehospitalization rates of patients recently discharged on a regimen of risperidone or clozapine. *Am J Psychiatry* 156, 863–8.

Csernansky J, Okamoto A (1999). Risperidone vs

haloperidol for prevention of relapse in schizophrenia and schizoaffective disorders: a long-term double-blind comparison. Poster presented at the 12th Congress of the European College of Neuropsychopharmacology, London, 21–25 September 1999.

Davies A, Langley PC, Keks NA, et al (1998). Risperidone versus haloperidol: II. Cost-effectiveness. *Clin Ther* **20**, 196–213.

Davies LM, Drummond MF (1993). Assessment of costs and benefits of drug therapy for treatment-resistant schizophrenia in the United Kingdom. *Br J Psychiatry* **162**, 38–42.

Del Paggio D, Douglas S (1998). The pharmacoeconomics and efficacy of atypical antipsychotics within Alameda County BHCS. *Behav Health Care* **2**, 10–14.

Drew LR, Hodgson DM, Griffiths KM (1999). Clozapine in community practice: a 3-year follow-up study in the Australian Capital Territory. *Aust NZ J Psychiatry* **33**, 667–75.

Drummond MF, Knapp MRJ, Burns TP, et al (1998). Issues in the design of studies for the economic evaluation of new atypical antipsychotics: the ESTO study. *J Ment Health Policy Econ* **1**, 15–22.

Edgell ET, Hamilton SH, Revicki DA, et al (1998). Costs of olanzapine treatment compared with haloperidol for schizophrenia: results from a randomized clinical trial. Poster presented at the 21st CINP Congress, Glasgow, July 1998.

Edgell ET, Hamilton SH, Gregor KJ (1999). Functional outcomes in schizophrenia: a European comparison of olanzapine and haloperidol (abstract). Poster presented at the 12th Congress of the European College of Neuropsychopharmacology, London, 21–25 September 1999.

Essock SM, Hargreaves WA, Dohm FA, et al

(1996). Clozapine eligibility among State hospital patients. *Schizophr Bull* **22**, 15–25.

Finley PR, Sommer BR, Corbitt JL, et al (1998). Risperidone: clinical outcome predictors and cost-effectiveness in a naturalistic setting. *Psychopharmacol Bull* **34**, 75–81.

Fitton A, Benfield P (1993). Clozapine: an appraisal of its pharmacoeconomic benefits in the treatment of schizophrenia. *Pharmacoeconomics* **4**, 131–56.

Frankenburg FR, Zanarini MC, Cole JO, et al (1992). Hospitalization rates among clozapine-treated patients: a prospective cost-benefit analysis. *Ann Clin Psychiatry* **4**, 247–50.

Geronimi-Ferret D, Lesay M, Barges-Bertocchio MH (1997). Medico-economic evaluation of treatment with clozapine versus treatment with previous neuroleptics. *Encephale* **23** (spec. no. 4), 24–31.

Ghaemi SN, Ziegler DM, Peachey TJ, et al (1998). Cost-effectiveness of clozapine therapy for severe psychosis. *Psychiatr Serv* **49**, 829–31.

Ginsberg G, Shani S, Lev B (1998). Cost-benefit analysis of risperidone and clozapine in the treatment of schizophrenia in Israel. *Pharmacoeconomics* **13**, 231–41.

Grainger DL, Hamilton SH, Genduso LA, et al (1998a). Medical resource use and work and social outcomes for olanzapine compared with haloperidol in the treatment of schizophrenia and other psychotic disorders. Poster presented at the 21st Congress of the CINP, Glasgow, July 1998.

Grainger DL, Edgell ET, Andersen SW (1998b). Resource use and quality of life of olanzapine compared with risperidone: results from an international randomized clinical trial. Abstract presented at 11th European College of Neuropsychopharmacology Congress, Paris, 31 October–4 November 1998.

Gregor K, Gureje O, Lambert T, et al (1999). Olanzapine versus risperidone in the management of schizophrenia: a randomized double-blind study in Australia and New Zealand. Abstract presented at the XIth World Congress of Psychiatry, Hamburg, 6–11 August 1999.

Guest JF, Hart WM. Cookson RF, et al (1996). Pharmacoeconomic evaluation of long-term treatment with risperidone for patients with chronic schizophrenia. *Br J Med Econ* **10**, 59–67.

Gury C, Dechelette N, Gayral P (1996). Leponex: experience of the hospital pharmacist. *Encephale* **3**, 61–5.

Hamilton SH, Revicki DA, Genduso LA, et al (1998). Costs of olanzapine treatment compared with haloperidol for schizophrenia: results from a randomized clinical trial (abstract). Poster presented at the American Psychiatric Association Annual Meeting, Toronto, 1998.

Hamilton SH, Revicki DA, Edgell ET, et al (1999). Clinical and economic outcomes of olanzapine compared with haloperidol for schizophrenia: results from a randomised clinical trial. *Pharmacoeconomics* **15**, 469–80.

Hammond CM, Pierson JF, Grande TP, et al (1999). Economic evaluation of risperidone in an outpatient population. *Ann Pharmacother* **33**, 1160–6.

Hellewell JSE, Kalali AH, Langham SJ, et al (1999). Patient satisfaction and acceptability of long-term treatment with quetiapine. *Int J Psychiatry Clin Pract* **3**, 105–13.

Honigfeld G, Patin J (1990). A two-year clinical and economic follow-up of patients on clozapine. *Hosp Community Psychiatry* **41**, 882–5.

Jonsson D, Wålinder J (1995). Cost-effectiveness of clozapine treatment in therapy-refractory schizophrenia. *Acta Psychiatr Scand* **92**, 199–201.

Keks NA (1997). Impact of newer antipsychotics on outcomes in schizophrenia. *Clin Ther* **19**, 148–58.

Lee KMS, Langham SJ, Graves N, et al (1998). Health economic audit of long-term treatment with 'Seroquel' for patients with chronic schizophrenia. Poster presented at the European College of Neuropharmacology, 1998.

Le Pen C, Lilliu H, Allicar MP, et al (1999). Comparaison économique de l'olanzapine *versus* halopéridol dans le traitement de la schizophrénie en France. *Encéphale* **25**, 281–6.

Malla AK (1998). Outcome in schizophrenia: a comparison of treatment with risperidone and typical antipsychotics. Poster presented at the 151st Annual Meeting of the American Psychiatric Association, Toronto, 30 May–4 June 1998.

Matheson LA, Cook HM, McKenna P, et al (1994). Value for money care for patients with schizophrenia. *Br J Med Econ* **7**, 25–34.

Maynard A, Bloor K (1998). Building castles on sands or quicksands? *Br J Psychiatry* **173**, 12–18.

Meltzer HY, Cola P, Way L, et al (1995). Cost effectiveness of clozapine in neuroleptic-resistant schizophrenia. *Am J Psychiatry* **150**, 1630–8.

Moore DB, Kelly DL, Sherr JD, et al (1998). Rehospitalization rates for depot antipsychotics and pharmacoeconomic implications: comparison with risperidone. *Am J Health Syst Pharm* **55** (suppl. 4), 17–19.

Morris S, Hogan T, McGuire A (1998). The cost-effectiveness of clozapine: a survey of the literature. *Clin Drug Invest* **15**, 137–52.

Nightengale BS, Crumly JM, Liao J, et al (1998). Economic outcomes of antipsychotic agents in a medicaid population: traditional gents vs risperidone. *Psychopharmac Bull* **34**, 373–82.

Palmer CS, Revicki DA, Genduso LA, et al (1998). A cost-effectiveness clinical decision analysis model for schizophrenia. *Am J Managed Care* **4**, 345–55.

Percudani M, Fattore G, Galletta J, et al (1999). Health care costs of therapy-refractory schizophrenic patients treated with clozapine: a study in a community psychiatric service in Italy. *Acta Psychiatr Scand* **99**, 274–80.

Pollack S, Woerner MG, Howard A, et al (1998). Clozapine reduces rehospitalization among schizophrenia patients. *Psychopharmacol Bull* **34**, 89–92.

Procyshyn RM, Zerjav S (1998). Drug utilization patterns and outcomes associated with in-hospital treatment with risperidone or olanzapine. *Clin Ther* **20**, 1203–17.

Reid WH (1999). New vs. old antipsychotics: the Texas Experience. *J Clin Psychiatry* **60** (suppl. 1), 23–5.

Reid WH, Mason M (1998). Psychiatric hospital utilization in patients treated with clozapine for up to 4.5 years in a State mental health care system. *J Clin Psychiatry* **59**, 189–94.

Reid WH, Mason M, Toprac M (1994). Savings in hospital bed-days related to treatment with clozapine. *Hosp Community Psychiatry* **45**, 261–4.

Revicki DA (1999). Pharmacoeconomic evaluation of treatments for refractory schizophrenia:

clozapine-related studies. *J Clin Psychiatry* **60** (suppl. 1), 7–11.

Revicki DA, Luce BR, Weschler JM et al (1990). Cost-effectiveness of clozapine for treatment-resistant schizophrenic patients. *Hosp Community Psychiatry* **41**, 850–69.

Robert G, Kennedy P (1997). Establishing cost-effectiveness of atypical neuroleptics. *Br J Psychiatry* **171**, 103–4.

Rosenheck R, Cramer J, Xu W, et al (1997). A comparison of clozapine and haloperidol in hospitalized patients with refractory schizophrenia. *N Engl J Med* **337**, 809–15.

Sacristán JA, Gómez JC, Martin J, et al (1998). Pharmacoeconomic assessment of olanzapine in the treatment of refractory schizophrenia based on a pilot clinical study. *Clin Drug Invest* **15**, 29–35.

Sacristan JA, Gómez JC, Salvador-Carulla L (1997). Análisis coste-efectividad de olanzapina frente a haloperidol en el tratamiento de la esquizofrenia en España. *Actas Luso-Espan Neurol Psiqu Ciencias Afines* **25**, 225–34.

Schiller MJ, Shumway M, Hargreaves WA (1999). Treatment costs and patient outcomes with use of risperidone in a public mental health setting. *Psychiatr Serv* **50**, 228–32.

Souêtre E, Martin P, Lecanu JP, et al (1992). Valuation médico-économomique des neuroleptiques dans la schizophrénie. *Encéphale*, **18**, 263–9.

Spannheimer A, Clouth J (1999). Pharmacoeconomic evaluation of the treatment of schizophrenia in Germany: a comparison of olanzapine and haloperidol. Poster presented at the 12th Congress of the European College of Neuropsychopharmacology, London, 21–25 September 1999.

Spannheimer A, Clouth J, Gregor KJ (1999). Pharmacoeconomic evaluation of the treatment of schizophrenia in Germany: a comparison of olanzapine, risperidone and haloperidol using a clinical decision model. Poster presented at the ISPOR Second Annual European Meeting, Edinburgh, November 1999.

Thompson D (1996). Costs of treatment with risperidone and clozapine. Poster presented at the American Psychiatric Association Annual Meeting, New York, May 1996.

Tollefson GD, Beasley CM, Tran PV (1997). Olanzapine versus haloperidol in the treatment of schizophrenia and schizoaffective and schizophreniform disorders: results of an international collaborative trial. *Am J Psychiatry* **154**, 457–65.

Tran PV, Hamilton SH, Kuntz AJ, et al (1997). Double-blind comparison of olanzapine versus risperidone in the treatment of schizophrenia and other psychotic disorders. *J Clin Psychopharmacol* **17**, 407–18.

Tunis SL, Croghan TW, Heilman DK, et al (1998). Changes in perceived physical and mental health status of a schizophrenia patient population following initiation of a conventional or an atypical antipsychotic medication. Poster presented at the American Psychiatric Association Annual Meeting, Toronto, June 1998.

Viale G, Mechling L, Maislin G, et al (1997). Impact of risperidone on the use of mental health care resources. *Psychiatr Serv* **48**, 1153–9.

Weiss MA, McCollum M (1998). Cost impact of using olanzapine at a Veterans Affairs Medical Center. Poster presentation at the Third Annual Meeting of ISPOR, Philadelphia, May 1998. Abstract published in *Value Health* **1**, 25.

Wieselgren IM, Lindstrom E, Lindstrom L (1999). A cost-effectiveness clinical decision analysis for schizophrenia: results from Sweden. Poster presented at the 12th Congress of the European College of Neuropsychopharmacology, London, 21–25 September 1999.

Depression

John Donoghue

3

Depression is a common, serious, sometimes fatal illness that is 'chronic and recurrent in nature, impairs family life, reduces social adjustment, and is a burden on the community' (Klerman and Weissman, 1992). This disease chronicity magnifies both its societal impact and its economic burden. It has been estimated that more than 17% of the disability associated with mental disorders is the result of depressive disorders (Rosenbaum and Hylan, 1999), and that the global burden of depression, measured in terms of disability-adjusted life years, will rank second only to ischaemic heart disease by the year 2020 (Murray and Lopez, 1996).

Depression imposes a significant economic burden worldwide (Greenberg et al, 1993; Kind and Sorensen, 1993; Simon et al, 1995a; Rosenbaum and Hylan, 1999). It is associated with an increase in the use of all sectors of health-care provision, with disproportionately high costs. One study comparing over 6000 patients with depression with randomly selected control subjects showed markedly higher health-care costs in the depressed group for every component of health costs, and in every subset of patients (Simon et al, 1995a). These differences could not be accounted for by the use of specialist mental health services, nor by the costs of antidepressant medicines, and were maintained over a 12-month period, suggesting chronic, unremitting, disproportionate use of health-care resources by depressed patients (Simon et al, 1995a). A Swedish study found similar disproportionately high use of health-care resources (Bingefors et al, 1995). In a large primary-care study, 7% of patients were prescribed an antidepressant; they consumed 24% of all prescribed medicines, 14% of all hospital bed days, and 13% of all general practitioner visits.

Antidepressant medicines have a major role in the treatment of depression, and account for a significant proportion of health-care costs (Kind and Sorensen, 1992; Freemantle et al, 1993; Greenberg et al, 1993). The continuing development of antidepressant agents has increased the availability of newer drugs that have similar efficacy but are more expensive than the older antidepressants (Song et al, 1993). This chapter addresses the complex question of whether there is clear evidence that the use of any single antidepressant or group of antidepressants is more cost-effective than any other.

Types of cost

The costs associated with depression are complex and have been categorized as direct or indirect, and as health care or social care

(Kind and Sorenson, 1992). This discussion is limited to considerations of direct health-care costs only, i.e. the health-care costs related directly to the treatment of a depressed individual. On an empirical level it is tempting to assume that the use of more expensive drugs that are found in clinical trials to have efficacy similar to existing treatments may increase the cost of treatment (Freemantle et al, 1993; Song et al, 1993; Hotopf et al, 1996). However, this approach fails to take into account the complex interactions that take place between the treatment prescribed, the patient, and the system of health care in which the treatment is delivered. Pharmacoeconomic evaluations must address the question of what happens to patients following a drug intervention, and at what cost. Research methods should embrace all identifiable components of treatment and include clinical evaluations, epidemiology, economics, or a synthesis of these methods (Bootman, 1995).

Types of pharmacoeconomic analysis

Several analyses are open when considering pharmacoeconomic evaluations of antidepressants (Reeder, 1995; Malek, 1996). *Cost-minimization analysis* concerns a direct comparison only between treatments that produce identical outcomes. However, other than in the case of generic substitution, this is unlikely to occur in the real world. More frequently, economic evaluations revolve around complex alternatives which produce multiple and different outcomes. For this reason, *cost-effectiveness analysis* evaluates the costs and outcomes in actual use when different interventions are intended to produce similar outcomes but have different rates of success. *Cost-utility analysis* expresses the cost of outcomes in units of patient benefit, and has resulted in the development of concepts such as the quality-adjusted life year (QALY) (Murray and Lopez, 1996), which combines aspects of both quantity and quality of life as an outcome of treatment. This approach is uncommon in pharmacoeconomic considerations of the treatment of depression, although some studies (Hatziandreu et al, 1994; CCOHTA, 1997) have assigned cost-utility values (QALY) in decision analytic models. *Cost-benefit analyses* are rarely performed in mental health studies although they are very powerful techniques.

Evidence for differences in pharmacoeconomic outcomes

Data on antidepressant drugs are available from a number of sources: randomized, controlled clinical trials (RCTs) in both hospital and primary-care populations; decision analytic models; population-based naturalistic observational studies of usual

clinical practice; and naturalistic 'real world' studies which take place within the ambit of normal clinical practice but in which some of the variables are controlled.

The main focus of pharmacoeconomic studies of antidepressants has inevitably fallen on comparisons between tricyclic antidepressants (TCAs) and the more expensive selective serotonin reuptake inhibitors (SSRIs). Few data are available for comparisons within the SSRIs or for newer antidepressants.

Tricyclic antidepressants versus SSRIs

Data from controlled trials

Randomized, controlled clinical trials reduce bias and variability by a process of selection, randomization and standardization of treatment, and often take place under artificial conditions isolated from those of routine clinical practice (Freemantle et al, 1993; Simon et al, 1995b). Yet it is the *uncontrolled* interactions of a drug technology with patients, health-care workers and the system of health care that ultimately lead to much of the variability in outcomes and expenditures in clinical practice. Thus the value of RCTs in evaluating cost-effectiveness in clinical practice may be limited (Reeder, 1995; Simon et al, 1995b; Hotopf et al, 1996).

Clinical trials of antidepressants suggest

similar efficacy between individual antidepressants or groups of antidepressants (Song et al, 1993; Anderson and Tomenson, 1994; Geddes et al, 1999). It is tempting to infer from this that cheaper antidepressants must be more cost-effective, and indeed, this argument has been employed (Freemantle et al, 1993; Song et al, 1993; Hotopf et al, 1996). However, such a narrow focus fails to take into account either the recurrent or chronic nature of depressive illness or the complexities of delivering treatment. Such arguments involve cost minimization, not cost-effectiveness. Cost-minimization analyses of controlled trials cannot provide answers to questions of cost-effectiveness as they relate to clinical practice because there is no evidence that outcomes are replicated—or are even similar—in primary-care practice in heterogeneous populations. Indeed, the available evidence suggests that TCAs are rarely used effectively in clinical practice (Donoghue and Taylor, 2000).

Data from decision analytic models

Decision analytic models, or simulation models of clinical decision analysis, usually involve the creation of a treatment decision/outcome tree based on a synthesis of 'expert' opinion, sometimes using validated methods of canvassing opinion such as recruiting a Delphi panel (Hatziandreu et al, 1994; Einarson et al, 1995). The decision tree then uses data from RCTs in experiments that seek to simulate expected clinical practice. This methodology produces uncertain results. The models are based on assumptions about practice and outcomes in the absence of evidence for their validity, and as a consequence cannot lead to definitive conclusions (Freemantle et al, 1995; Hotopf et al, 1996). The resulting outcomes may not reflect clinical reality, not only because of the limitations of generalizing data from RCTs (Simon et al, 1995b), but also because under 'real world' conditions the behaviour of both clinicians and patients is variable. Models have yet to provide convincing evidence, and are most useful when a new drug is introduced into practice and there are no other data available on which to make any pharmacoeconomic assessment. They may also be useful in framing research questions or in informing the design of studies to investigate economic outcomes (Forder et al, 1996).

Decision analytic models have been constructed to compare the costs of TCAs with those of SSRIs and other compounds. These comparisons have included imipramine or amitriptyline versus paroxetine or sertraline (Stewart, 1994); imipramine versus paroxetine (Jonsson and Bebbington, 1994; McFarland, 1994; Lapierre et al, 1995); fluoxetine versus amitriptyline, clomipramine, doxepin and imipramine (Le Pen et al, 1994); venlafaxine versus amitriptyline, desipramine, imipramine, nortriptyline, fluoxetine, paroxetine, sertraline and trazodone (Einarson et al, 1995); venlafaxine versus SSRIs and TCAs (Einarson et al, 1997); imipramine versus nefazodone (Montgomery et al, 1996); citalopram versus amitriptyline, doxepin and trimipramine (Nuitjen et al, 1995); and SSRIs versus TCAs (CCOHTA, 1997).

With few exceptions, models find in favour of newer compounds (Jonsson and Bebbington, 1994; Le Pen et al, 1994; McFarland, 1994; Stewart, 1994; Einarson et al, 1995; Lapierre et al, 1995; Nuitjen et al, 1995; Montgomery et al, 1996). One study (CCOHTA, 1997) did make allowances for variations in practice and patient behaviour. The results indicated that in the short term treatment was likely to be more successful with an SSRI than with a TCA, but at a higher cost. However, when treatment drop-out rates found in naturalistic studies were substituted for drop-out rates found in controlled trials, the cost differences became smaller. When cost-utility analysis was applied, this increased cost was offset by improvements in quality of life for the patients.

Data from population-based studies

Naturalistic population-based studies use epidemiological methods to attempt to identify outcomes from 'real world' clinical practice in large, heterogeneous populations.

Such studies have inherent limitations in that the complex interactions of health-care systems result in the presence of interdependent variables whose influence on the outcomes is difficult or impossible to measure (Simon et al, 1995b). Common problems include selection bias, retrospective data collection, errors in data collection, and variability in the abilities and practice of physicians in primary-care settings (Donoghue and Tylee, 1996; Donoghue, 1998). There are also likely to be wide variations in physician and patient beliefs, expectations and behaviours, all of which may significantly alter the outcomes of treatment, for example the use of ineffective doses or premature discontinuation of treatment (Donoghue and Taylor, 2000). Despite these limitations, naturalistic studies (including both retrospective and prospective designs) may help to identify associations between antidepressant use and economic outcomes in the context of the health system in which the treatment was delivered, and offer the most generalizable results when treatments are applied in routine practice settings. Statistical techniques are emerging to reduce the influence of such unobserved factors (Forder et al, 1996; Hylan et al, 1997, 1998).

Naturalistic studies reveal that in primary care, the suboptimal use of antidepressants appears to be an almost universal practice worldwide. Patients treated with TCAs are much less likely to receive effective treatment than patients treated with SSRIs (Donoghue and Taylor, 2000). A longitudinal study of more than 16 000 patients found that patients prescribed an SSRI were at least 7 times more likely to complete 4 consecutive months of treatment at an effective dose than were patients prescribed a TCA (Dunn et al, 1999). Thus, despite the absence of direct pharmacoeconomic data, it appears unlikely that TCAs could prove more cost-effective than SSRIs because they are not used in ways known to be effective (Goldstein and Goodnick, 1998). These suggestions are supported by a study of the costs of treatment failure in a large Medicaid population, which found that treatment failure resulted in an increase in consumption of health resources to the value of US $1000 (1990 value) (McCombs et al, 1990). Such studies illustrate the important differences between the ways drugs are used in controlled trials and clinical practice. However, they fail to answer the question whether the *effective* use of TCAs would be more cost-effective than the use of SSRIs.

Naturalistic, retrospective database studies, which have set out specifically to investigate pharmacoeconomic outcomes, have included analyses of:

- health costs relating only to the treatment of depression (Sclar et al, 1994; Skaer et al, 1995, 1996)

- total direct health-care treatment expenditures (Croghan et al, 1997; Melton et al, 1997; Revicki et al, 1997; Crown et al, 1998; Hylan et al, 1998)
- absenteeism and work loss costs (Beuzen et al, 1993; Tollefson et al, 1993)

The consistent finding across different systems for delivering health care is that the costs for patients beginning treatment with an SSRI are equal to or lower than costs for patients who begin therapy with a TCA (Rosenbaum and Hylan, 1999). The higher acquisition costs of SSRIs tend to be offset by reduced consumption of other resources, including lower expenditures for hospitalizations and physician consultations.

Naturalistic 'real world' prospective studies

Another approach uses a synthesis of RCTs and naturalistic studies, while addressing the limitations of both (Simon et al, 1995b; Hotopf et al, 1996). In such studies the treatment setting is routine primary-care clinical practice; selection criteria are limited to those affecting safety; and treatment is 'normal', i.e. provided under conditions where differences in clinical practice and patient behaviour can emerge freely. However, participants are randomized to initial treatment, and accurate diagnosis and baseline assessments are recorded. This approach is thought to provide the means of reducing bias, reducing sources of error, and obtaining accurate data on cost-effectiveness.

Retrospective quasi-experimental study

The only study conducted in the UK (Forder et al, 1996) employed a retrospective, 'quasi-experimental' design in which patients from an open-label study of sertraline were compared with age- and gender-matched patients prescribed TCAs in a primary care setting. The study found that sertraline was more effective than TCAs (87% versus 74%, $p < 0.01$) and also more cost-effective, mainly because of the higher number of hospital admissions in the TCA group. This study had limitations in that patients prescribed TCAs were not randomly selected, a quarter of the patients in the TCA group failed to receive an effective dose, and objective measurements of outcome were not employed. Multivariate analysis suggested that despite the methodological limitations of the study, the differences in cost were due to the treatment received, and not to differences in patient characteristics. This study provides the first, albeit tentative, evidence of superior cost-effectiveness for SSRIs over TCAs in the UK.

Real-world controlled trial

To address the limitations inherent in both controlled and observational studies, Simon and colleagues developed a study design incorporating randomization of treatment and an intention-to-treat analysis into a prospective trial of 'normal' clinical practice (Simon et al, 1995b, 1996). This they dubbed a 'real world' study. Methodologically, it seems the least impaired study design, and is deserving of our attention. The primary purpose was to investigate whether an *initial* trial of treatment with a TCA would reduce overall treatment costs (Simon et al, 1996). A total of 536 patients were recruited from a health maintenance organization (HMO), and randomized to receive an initial prescription for desipramine, imipramine or fluoxetine, the only exclusion being a contraindication to any of the trial compounds; subsequent treatment was at the discretion of the primary-care physician. Fluoxetine showed several clinical advantages over the TCAs: more patients randomized to receive fluoxetine continued with the original treatment (80%) than patients prescribed either desipramine (52%) or imipramine (57%) ($p < 0.001$). More patients completed 90 days of treatment with fluoxetine (61%) compared with either desipramine (49%) or imipramine (48%) ($p < 0.02$). Fewer patients on fluoxetine (9%) discontinued treatment as a result of adverse effects, compared with desipramine (27%) or imipramine (28%) ($p < 0.001$). After 6 months there were no clinical differences between the groups, and although treatment costs were lowest for fluoxetine (US $1967) compared with desipramine (US $2361) or imipramine (US $2105) these differences were not statistically significant. Although it is tempting to infer that the study showed that an *initial* trial of treatment with a TCA failed to reduce overall treatment costs, this may have been the result of potential confounders in the study. The freedom to switch from one treatment to another, coupled with the intention-to-treat analysis, may have introduced a design bias in favour of the TCAs. Many of the patients randomized to initial treatment with a TCA subsequently switched treatment (desipramine 48%, imipramine 43%), two-thirds of them to fluoxetine. In contrast, only 20% of those initially randomized to fluoxetine switched, 46% of them to a TCA. Previous studies (Sclar et al, 1994; Skaer et al, 1995) suggested that this would produce changes across several interdependent variables including the costs of the drug, primary-care physician visits, out-patient psychiatric care, and in-patient costs both in general medicine and psychiatry. Switching between treatments and applying an intention-to-treat analysis may have disproportionately favoured the TCAs. A secondary analysis of treatment completers also found no significant difference in clinical outcome, and the authors acknowledged that this might have been a consequence of the large numbers of patients switching treatment, and that the compensating differences in the costs of general health resource consumption might have been chance findings (Simon et al, 1996).

Other issues

Pharmacoeconomic comparisons of SSRIs

Differences exist in primary care between the patterns of prescribing fluoxetine, paroxetine or sertraline, which may influence cost outcomes. Sertraline-treated patients are more likely to have their dose increased (Sclar et al, 1995; Donoghue, 1998), and to drop out of treatment prematurely (Donoghue, 1998). The apparent need to titrate doses upwards with sertraline may require more involvement by the clinician and may delay response to treatment, with resultant increases in direct health costs (Sclar et al, 1995). However, these economic findings are retrospective, may suffer from selection bias, and being derived from HMO patients may not be generalizable to other populations; confirmation in further studies is required.

New antidepressants

Apart from decision analytic models, pharmacoeconomic data for newer antidepressants are lacking.

Antidepressants versus psychotherapy

Various forms of psychotherapy are regarded as effective interventions in mild to moderate depression, but studies comparing the economics of psychotherapy and pharmacotherapy are few (Rosenbaum and Hylan, 1999). One study found that the total health-care costs for patients who received psychotherapy were no different from those for patients who received an antidepressant. However, no efficacy measure was used (Edgell and Hylan, 1997). A randomized, prospective study which evaluated the treatment of depression with nortriptyline, interpersonal therapy or treatment as usual, with outcomes expressed in quality-adjusted life years, found that nortriptyline but not interpersonal therapy was a cost-effective alternative to treatment as usual (Lave et al, 1998).

Systems for delivering health care

Outcomes of treatment in primary care depend on a complex set of interactions between the treatment offered, the practice of health-care professionals, the behaviour of patients, and the system of health care in which the treatment is delivered. The practice of health-care professionals and the behaviour of patients may be influenced by culture and training. Even where cultural norms,

expectations and training are similar, differences in the delivery of health care may influence outcomes. There may be different processes for making decisions, different costs and different criteria for determining what treatment may be offered. For example, in the USA, care provided by an HMO or care provided by Medicaid may be delivered differently. Similarly, in the UK, care provided in the National Health Service may be subject to different pressures and constraints from care provided in the private sector. It is likely that pharmacoeconomic findings are specific to the system of health care in which a study is conducted and are not generalizable to other systems of care.

Comment

The evidence that any one antidepressant or group of antidepressant drugs provides more cost-effective treatment than any other remains inconclusive. Several studies (Sclar et al, 1994, 1995; Bingefors et al, 1995; Simon et al, 1995a, b, 1996; Skaer et al, 1995; Forder et al, 1996; Hylan et al, 1997) have described the breadth of health utilization that needs to be included for pharmacoeconomic studies. Nevertheless, attempts are still being made to limit the broad perspective that is required. Hotopf et al (1996) suggested that data for pharmacoeconomic evaluations should be limited to three sources: randomized, controlled trials; meta-analyses;

and controlled trials of cost-effectiveness. However, such studies may underestimate the complexities of practice in the real world where patients are not randomized and outcomes are not measured as a point on a rating scale.

There is compelling evidence that older TCAs are not used effectively (Donoghue and Taylor, 2000), and this may result in treatment failure and a disproportionately higher consumption of health resources by patients prescribed these drugs (McCombs et al, 1990; Bingefors et al, 1995; Simon et al, 1995a). To date, the limited evidence is consistently in one direction: SSRIs are at best more cost-effective than TCAs (Sclar et al, 1994; Skaer et al, 1995; Forder et al, 1996) or at worst cost-neutral (Simon et al, 1996). However, these findings are from populations that may not be generalizable, and may be subject to selection bias. A constant caveat must be the knowledge that it is probably unsafe to generalize findings from one system of health care to another, where different health policies determine service structures, services vary, referral to specialist services is based on different criteria, and cost structures for drugs and services may be very different.

It is essential that research to assess the cost-effectiveness of antidepressant pharmacotherapy continues and that better pharmacoeconomic research methods evolve. Naturalistic studies may be used to observe how antidepressant drugs perform in practice,

to frame the questions that need to be addressed in controlled studies to identify differences if and where they exist. In the absence of conclusive evidence for superior cost-effectiveness for any one antidepressant, the problem of inadequate treatment is economically more important than the question of differential cost-effectiveness between antidepressants. The emphasis should be on optimizing the effectiveness with which antidepressants are used, and this seems unlikely to be achieved if primacy is given to TCAs because of their lower acquisition cost.

References

Anderson IM, Tomenson BM (1994). The efficacy of selective serotonin reuptake inhibitors in depression: a meta-analysis of studies against tricyclic antidepressants. *J Psychopharmacol* 8, 238–49.

Beuzen JN, Ravily VF, Soutre EF, Thomander L (1993). Impact of fluoxetine on work loss in depression. *Int Clin Psychopharmacol*, 8, 319–21.

Bingefors KAL, Isacson DGL, von Knorring L, Smedby B (1995). Prescription drug and healthcare use among Swedish patients treated with antidepressants. *Ann Pharmacother* 29, 566–72.

Bootman JL (1995). Pharmacoeconomics and outcomes research. *Am J Health Syst Pharm* 52 (suppl. 3), S16–19.

[CCOHTA] Canadian Coordinating Office for Health Technology Assessment (1997). *Selective Serotonin Re-uptake Inhibitors (SSRIs) for Major Depression*, Part II: *The Cost-*

effectiveness of SSRIs in the Treatment of Depression. Ottowa: CCOHTA.

Croghan TW, Lair TJ, Engelhart LE, et al (1997). Effect of antidepressant therapy on health care utilization and costs in primary care. *Psychiatr Serv* **48**, 1420–6.

Crown WH, Hylan TR, Meneades L (1998). Antidepressant selection and use and health care expenditures: an empirical approach. *Pharmacoeconomics* **13**, 435–48.

Donoghue JM (1998). Selective serotonin re-uptake inhibitor use in primary care: a five year naturalistic study. *Clin Drug Invest* **16**, 453–62.

Donoghue JM, Tylee A (1996). The treatment of depression: prescribing patterns of antidepressants in primary care in the United Kingdom. *Br J Psychiatry* **168**, 164–8.

Donoghue JM, Taylor DM (2000). Suboptimal use of antidepressants in the treatment of depression. *CNS Drugs* **13**, 365–83.

Dunn RL, Donoghue JM, Ozminkowski RJ, et al (1999). Longitudinal patterns of antidepressant prescribing in primary care in the UK: comparison with treatment guidelines. *J Psychopharmacol* **13**, 136–43.

Edgell ET, Hylan TR (1997). Economic outcomes associated with initial treatment choice in depression: a retrospective database analysis. *Am J Managed Care* **3**, S51.

Einarson TR, Arikian S, Sweeney S, Doyle J (1995). A model to evaluate the cost effectiveness of oral therapies in the management of patients with major depressive disorders. *Clin Ther* **17**, 136–53.

Forder J, Kavanagh S, Fenyo A (1996). A comparison of the cost-effectiveness of sertraline versus tricyclic antidepressants in primary care. *J Affective Disord* **38**, 97–111.

Freemantle N, Long A, Mason J, et al (1993). The treatment of depression in primary care. *Effective Health Care* **5**, 1–12.

Freemantle N, House A, Mason J, Song F, Sheldon T (1995). Economics of treatment of depression [letter]. *Br J Psychiatry* **166**, 397.

Geddes JR, Freemantle N, Mason J, Eccles MP, Boynton J (1999). SSRIs versus alternative antidepressants in depressive disorder (Cochrane Review). In: *Cochrane Library*, Issue 4. Oxford: Update Software.

Goldstein BJ, Goodnick PJ (1998). Selective serotonin reuptake inhibitors in the treatment of affective disorders – III. Tolerability, safety and pharmacoeconomics. *J Psychopharmacol* **12** (suppl. B), S55–87.

Greenberg PE, Stiglin LE, Finkelstein SN, Bendt ER (1993). The economic burden of depression in 1990. *J Clin Psychiatry* **54**, 405–18.

Hatziandreu EJ, Brown RE, Revicki DA, et al (1994). Cost-utility of maintenance treatment of recurrent depression with sertraline versus episodic treatment with dothiepin. *Pharmacoeconomics* **5**, 249–64.

Hotopf M, Lewis G, Normand C (1996). Are SSRIs a cost effective alternative to tricyclics? *Br J Psychiatry* **168**, 404–9.

Hylan TR, Neslusan CA, Baldridge RM, et al (1997). Selective serotonin reuptake inhibitor antidepressant selection and anxiolytic and sedative hypnotic prescribing: a multivariate analysis. *J Clin Outcomes Manage* **4**, 16–22.

Hylan TR, Crown WH, Meneades L, et al (1998). SSRI and TCA antidepressant selection and health care costs: a multivariate analysis. *J Affective Disord* **47**, 71–9.

Jonsson B, Bebbington PE (1994). What price depression? The cost of depression and the cost-effectiveness of pharmacological treatment. *Br J Psychiatry* **164**, 665–73.

Kind P, Sorensen J (1993). The costs of depression. *Int Clin Psychopharmacol* 7, 191–5.

Klerman GL, Weissman MM (1992). The course, morbidity, and costs of depression. *Arch Gen Psychiatry* **49**, 831–4.

Lapierre Y, Bentkover J, Schainbaum S, Manners S (1995). Direct cost of depression: analysis of treatment costs of paroxetine versus imipramine in Canada. *Can J Psychiatry* **40**, 370–7.

Lave JR, Frank RG, Shulberg HC, Kamlet MS (1998). Cost-effectiveness of treatments for major depression in primary care practice. *Arch Gen Psychiatry* **55**, 645–51.

Le Pen C, Levy E, Ravily J, et al (1994). The cost of treatment dropout in depression. A cost-benefit analysis of fluoxetine vs tricyclics. *J Affective Disord* **31**, 1–18.

Malek M (1996). Pharmacoeconomics: (1) Introduction. *Pharm J* **256**, 759–61.

McCombs JS, Nichol MB, Stimmel GL, et al (1990). The cost of antidepressant drug therapy failure: a study of antidepressant use patterns in a Medicaid population. *J Clin Psychiatry* **51** (6, suppl.), 60–9.

McFarland BH (1994). Cost-effectiveness considerations for managed care systems: treating depression in primary care. *Am J Med* **97** (suppl. 6A), 47–58S.

Melton ST, Kirkwood CK, Farrar TW, et al (1997). Economic evaluation of paroxetine and imipramine in depressed outpatient. *Psychopharmacol Bull* **33**, 93–100.

Montgomery SA, Brown R, Clark M (1996). Economic analysis of treating depression with nefazodone v. imipramine. *Br J Psychiatry* **168**, 768–71.

Murray CJ, Lopez AD (1996). *The Global Burden of Disease*. Geneva: World Health Organization.

Nuitjen MJC, Hardens M, Souetre E (1995). A Markov Process Analysis comparing the cost effectiveness of maintenance therapy with citalopram versus standard therapy in major depression. *Pharmacoeconomics* **8**, 159–68.

Reeder CE (1995). Overview of pharmacoeconomics and pharmaceutical outcomes evaluations. *Am J Health Syst Pharm* **52** (suppl. 3), S5–8.

Revicki DA, Palmer CS, Phillips SD, et al (1997). Acute medical costs of fluoxetine versus tricyclic antidepressants: a prospective multicentre study of antidepressant drug overdoses. *Pharmacoeconomics* **11**, 48–55.

Rosenbaum JF, Hylan TR (1999). Costs of depressive disorders: a review. In: Maj M, Sartorius N, eds, World Psychiatric Association Series Evidence and Experience in Psychiatry, Volume 1: *Depressive Disorders*. Chichester: John Wiley.

Sclar DA, Robison LM, Skaer TL et al (1994). Antidepressant pharmacotherapy: economic outcomes in a Health Maintenance Organisation. *Clin Ther* **16**, 715–30.

Sclar DA, Robison LM, Skaer TL, et al (1995). Antidepressant pharmacotherapy: economic evaluation of fluoxetine, paroxetine and sertraline in a health maintenance organisation. *J Int Med Res* **23**, 395–412.

Simon GE, VonKorff M, Barlow W (1995a). Health care costs of primary care patients with recognised depression. *Arch Gen Psychiatry* **52**, 850–6.

Simon G, Wagner E, VonKorff M (1995b). Cost-effectiveness comparisons using 'Real World' randomised trials: the case of new antidepressant drugs. *J Clin Epidemiol* **48**, 363–73.

Simon GE, VonKorff M, Heiligenstein JH, et al
(1996). Initial antidepressant choice in
primary care. *JAMA* **275**, 1897–902.

Skaer TL, Sclar DA, Robison LM, et al (1995).
Economic valuation of amitriptyline,
desipramine, nortriptyline, and sertraline in
the management of patients with depression.
Curr Ther Res **56**, 556–67.

Skaer TL, Sclar DA, Robison LM, et al (1996).
Antidepressant pharmacotherapy: effect on
women's resource utilization within a health
maintenance organization. *Appl Ther* **1**,
45–52.

Song F, Freemantle N, Sheldon T, et al (1993).
Selective serotonin reuptake inhibitors: meta-
analysis of efficacy and acceptability. *Br Med J*
306, 683–7.

Stewart A (1994). Antidepressant pharmacotherapy:
cost comparison of SSRIs and TCAs. *Br J
Med Econ* **7**, 67–79.

Tollefson GD, Souetre E, Thomander L, Potvin JH
(1993). Comorbid anxious signs and
symptoms in major depression: impact on
functional work capacity and comparative
treatment outcomes. *Int Clin Psychopharmacol*
8, 281–93.

Anxiety disorders

Malcolm Lader

4

Cost-containment policies throughout the world are forcing health-care managers, providers, doctors and other professionals to consider the cost of treatment as well as its clinical efficacy and safety. Those responsible for allocating health-care resources need to prioritize in order to maximize the health gain from any given budget. Economic evaluation with its methods such as cost-benefit analysis, cost-effectiveness analysis, cost-utility analysis and marginal analysis has opened up new perspectives on this area. In return, clinicians have had to reanalyse the concepts of illness and health, resulting in measurements such as the quality-adjusted life year. Nowhere is this more difficult than in psychiatry, with its lack of precision in diagnosis, evaluation of treatment and prognosis.

The anxiety disorders are a case in point. They comprise a range of conditions contiguous with the affective disorders and the stress responses (Table 4.1). Much overlap and comorbidity exist. Furthermore, definitions and diagnostic criteria have changed substantially over the years. For example, generalized anxiety disorder is a rare condition in its 'pure' form, but a common condition if comorbid phobic and depressive disorders are accepted.

Table 4.1
The ICD–10 classification of anxiety disorders.

F40 **Phobic anxiety disorders**

  F40.0 *Agoraphobia*
     .00 Without panic disorder
     .01 With panic disorder
  F40.1 *Social phobias*
  F40.2 *Specific (isolated) phobias*
  F40.8 *Other phobic anxiety disorders*
  F40.9 *Phobic anxiety disorder, unspecified*

F41 **Other anxiety disorders**

  F41.0 *Panic disorder [episodic paroxysmal anxiety]*
  F41.1 *Generalized anxiety disorder*
  F41.2 *Mixed anxiety and depressive disorder*
  F41.3 *Other mixed anxiety disorders*
  F41.8 *Other specified anxiety disorders*
  F41.9 *Anxiety disorder, unspecified*

F42 **Obsessive–compulsive disorder**

  F42.0 *Predominantly obsessional thoughts or ruminations*
  F42.1 *Predominantly compulsive acts [obsessional rituals]*
  F42.2 *Mixed obsessional thoughts and acts*
  F42.8 *Other obsessive–compulsive disorders*
  F42.9 *Obsessive–compulsive disorder, unspecified*

F43 **Reaction to severe stress, and adjustment disorders**

  F43.0 *Acute stress reaction*
  F43.1 *Post-traumatic stress disorder*
  F43.2 *Adjustment disorders*
     .20 Brief depressive reaction
     .21 Prolonged depressive reaction
     .22 Mixed anxiety and depressive reaction
     .23 With predominant disturbance of other emotions
     .24 With predominant disturbance of conduct
     .25 With mixed disturbance of emotions and conduct
     .28 With other specified predominant symptoms
  F43.8 *Other reactions to severe stress*
  F43.9 *Reaction to severe stress, unspecified*

A further factor concerns the milieu in which the anxiety disorders are encountered. These are essentially detected, diagnosed and treated by primary-care practitioners. In the UK, for instance, less than 10% of such cases are referred to specialists, although the figure tends to be higher in the USA and continental Europe. General practitioners often make syndromal or even symptomatic assessments rather than diagnosing disorders, so it may be difficult to extrapolate across countries.

Shah and Jenkins (2000) in a review of mental health economic studies from around the world identified 40 cost-of-illness studies, of which five covered all disorders, one neuroses, two panic disorders and one anxiety. All were from developed countries. There were numerous cost-effectiveness studies but none involving the anxiety disorders specifically. One study in the UK examined the cost-benefit analysis of a controlled trial of nurse therapy for neurosis in primary care (Ginsberg et al, 1984).

In this chapter pharmacoeconomic considerations of the anxiety disorders in general are outlined, followed by accounts of some studies in each major disorder.

Anxiety disorders

To reach agreed criteria, anxiety disorders must cause significant distress or interference with the patient's life, leading to significant personal costs. Symptoms alone are insufficient for a diagnosis. In addition, these disorders impose direct and indirect costs on society through the medical resources devoted to their diagnosis, treatment and rehabilitation, and reduced or lost productivity.

Anxiety disorders are very common. A survey in the USA indicated that about a quarter of the adult population suffered from at least one anxiety disorder during their lifetime (Kessler et al, 1994). Another study, the US Epidemiologic Catchment Area (ECA) programme, enumerated 6.4 million persons with anxiety disorders who made 98 million visits to their doctors in a 1-year period (Narrow et al, 1993). Eighty per cent of these visits were for phobic disorders (5.2 million persons; 15.1 visits per person per year). Panic disorders accounted for 1.1 million (18.6 visits) and obsessive–compulsive disorders for 1.5 million persons (20.9 visits). These figures for health-care utilization are in the same range as those for schizophrenia (16.0 visits) and affective disorder (18.0 visits). People with phobic disorders tended to make greater use of emergency departments (13.1 visits per patient per year) than the total anxiety disorder population (4.4 visits).

Data from the ECA were used in an analysis of the social costs of anxiety disorders (Leon et al, 1995). Financial dependence was high among anxious individuals, particularly those with panic disorders (unemployment among men was 60%). Chronic unemployment was also several times more common than in the general population.

Further detailed analyses of the ECA data have been extrapolated to USA national costs (Rice and Miller, 1998). It was calculated that the economic costs of mental disorders in 1990 in the USA totalled US$147.8 billion. Anxiety disorders were the most costly, amounting to $46.6 billion, just under a third of the total. Direct costs spent on mental health care totalled $67 billion, of which anxiety disorders accounted for only $11 billion (16.5%). Drug costs were $2191 million, of which anxiety disorders accounted for $1167 million—over half. Morbidity costs—the value of goods and services not produced because of mental disorders – amounted to $63.1 billion, with anxiety disorders accounting for $34.2 billion, 54.2% of the total. This reflects the high prevalence of anxiety disorders in the community and the high associated rate of lost productivity. In contrast, patients with affective disorders appeared better able to function (Rice and Miller, 1995). In summary, anxiety disorders are common, disruptive and costly to society; drug treatment is a substantial element of treatment costs (11%) compared with, say, schizophrenia (2.2%).

Another study used data from the National Comorbidity Study (Greenberg et al, 1999). The annual economic burden of anxiety disorders was estimated at US$42.3 billion in 1990 terms. This represents an annual cost

per sufferer of $1542, and a cost to the workplace of $256 per suffering worker, mostly attributed to lowered productivity rather than absenteeism. By far the largest item (54% of the total) was non-psychiatric direct medical costs. Direct psychiatric costs were 31%. Detailed cost-of-illness estimation is tabulated. Direct pharmaceutical costs were about $750 million. Post-traumatic stress disorder and panic disorder were the anxiety disorders with the highest rates of service use.

Extrapolation to other countries is not easy. Canada has a very different health-care system to the USA. A small-scale study involving 466 anxiety disorder patients in Quebec established a clear relationship between the severity of the disorder and utilization of health services (McCusker et al, 1997). Patients with obsessive–compulsive disorder were particularly likely to seek treatment. No information on drug use was presented.

Cost-effectiveness of treatment

Treating a condition is usually cheaper than not treating it (the offset effect). A Spanish study of panic disorder patients reported an offset effect of 14% following 12 months of drug treatment (Salvador-Carulla et al, 1995). Thus, the total direct costs of health-care use during the previous year and the year following diagnosis were US$29 000 and US$46 000 respectively, but the estimated indirect costs of lost productivity were about US$66 000 and US$14 000. The high indirect costs of the anxiety disorders result in high cost-effectiveness of efficacious treatments.

Out-patient treatment is substantially cheaper than in-patient management and is generally as effective (Lowman, 1991). A French study on patients with generalized anxiety disorder estimated costs per patient over 3 months to be US$423 for hospitalization, $335 for out-patient services and $43 for medications (Souetre et al, 1994). Comorbid conditions (mostly alcoholism and depression) doubled these direct health-care costs. Over three-quarters of all patients were taking anxiolytic medication.

Primary care studies

Evaluation of the economics of mental illness in primary care is an ongoing initiative of the UK Department of Health (Lloyd and Jenkins, 1995). A similar American study in Washington State included sub-threshold anxiety or depression, but these imposed relatively little economic load compared with disorder-level anxiety or depression (Simon et al, 1995). Mental health treatment accounted for only a small part of overall utilization, approximately 5%. Nevertheless, most patients with anxiety or depressive disorders showed considerable improvement. This was accompanied by only modest reductions in cost.

Specific disorders
Generalized anxiety disorder

The usually accepted prevalences for generalized anxiety disorder (GAD) are around 1.6% for current, 3.1% for 1 year and 5.1% lifetime (Roy-Byrne, 1996). The condition is twice as common in women as in men (Pigott, 1999). A small minority (10%) have GAD alone, and about the same proportion suffer from mixed anxiety and depression. Morbidity is high. About a half of those with uncomplicated GAD seek professional help, but two-thirds of those with comorbid GAD do so. Up to a half take medication at some point. The condition may coexist with other anxiety disorders such as phobias, with affective disorders, or with medical conditions such as unexplained chest pain and irritable bowel syndrome.

Generalized anxiety disorder has been relatively neglected from the point of view of both health economics and pharmacoeconomics. The changing diagnostic criteria have made it difficult to compare data over time, leading researchers to focus on the more clearly defined disorders such as panic and obsessions. Drug treatment has been dominated by the benzodiazepines, usually available generically and cheaply. However, as the final section of this chapter will show, all this is in flux.

Panic disorder

The lifetime prevalence rate for panic disorder is about 1.7%, divided into 2.4% in women, 1.0% in men. More people suffer panic attacks not reaching disorder level (4–10% of the population) (Katon, 1996). Patients with panic disorder make heavy demands of primary-care facilities and also emergency departments. In the USA, over a half of such patients have been hospitalized at some time. About a quarter are financially dependent and up to 10% are unable to seek work because of emotional problems (Katon, 1996). About 10% of patients with panic disorder are high health-care utilizers, accounting for 29% of primary-care visits, 52% of out-patient attendances, 48% of in-patient stays and 26% of prescriptions.

An Australian study compared medical utilization and costs in patients with panic disorder, those with social anxiety disorder, and a control group (Rees et al, 1998). Almost half of the panic disorder patients had seen a primary-care physician more than seven times over a 6-month period, compared with 7% of the social phobic patients and none of the control group. The mean costs were A$150, A$60 and A$20 respectively. The patients with panic disorder were treated with antidepressants (39%), benzodiazepines (15%), relaxants (12%), beta-blockers (7%) and other medication (7%). Twenty per cent received no medication. Patients with panic

disorder were likely to consult a specialist and incurred 5–6 times greater costs in this respect than socially phobic patients. Diagnostic tests for physical disorders were particularly high, averaging A$440, compared with A$20 for socially phobic or normal patients. Overall, the mean total direct cost estimates were: panic disorder A$1120, social phobia A$200 and normals A$100.

Unlike most anxiety disorders, panic disorder leads to a high utilization of general medical services, reflecting the frequency, severity and alarming nature of physical symptoms such as palpitations, gastrointestinal distress, respiratory problems and headaches (Zaubler and Katon, 1998). This can result in extensive investigations and sometimes inappropriate but expensive medications.

An earlier study yielded data at variance with these findings (Edlund and Swann, 1987). In a small group of patients with panic disorder, disability was marked: most reported a decreased quality of work and two-thirds claimed to have lost jobs or income. Half could not drive further than 5 kilometres and a third had increased their alcohol use. However, direct costs for treatment were not high, mainly because most had not sought treatment. Note that this study took place before panic disorder became generally recognized and publicized.

The Spanish study cited earlier (Salvador-Carulla et al, 1995) examined pharmaceutical costs. The costs before diagnosis for 61 patients were equivalent to US$3082 ($50 per patient); after diagnosis treatment comprising alprazolam and clomipramine cost in total US$11 631, an average of $190 per patient, nearly four times as much.

A major meta-analysis of treatment outcome was performed by Gould et al (1995). Forty-three studies were analysed, involving 76 interventions. Cognitive-behavioural treatments yielded the highest effect sizes (0.68), compared with pharmaceutical (0.47) and combination treatments (0.56). There was no significant difference ($p = 0.09$) between antidepressants (0.55) and benzodiazepines (0.40). The former drugs were associated with higher drop-out rates (25%) than the latter (13%). The lowest-cost interventions were imipramine and group cognitive-behavioural therapy at about US$600 per year. Low-dose (2.5 mg per day) alprazolam cost $1000 annually, high-dose alprazolam (6 mg per day) cost $1775, and fluoxetine cost $1875. However, each of these totals includes an item of $480 for session costs, so the cost of fluoxetine medication ($1400) is many times that of imipramine ($100).

Social anxiety disorder

The lifetime prevalence of social anxiety disorder is at least 2.5% and the condition often goes unrecognized (Nutt et al, 1999). Its economic impact is largely uncharted, but in view of its early onset and its stultification of educational, occupational and interpersonal development, the cost to society must be high (Ballenger et al, 1998). Conversely, medical costs—as quantified in the Australian study outlined above—are relatively modest (Rees et al, 1998). Comorbidity is an important factor in determining the type (and hence the cost) of treatment (Lecrubier, 1998). Thus people with uncomplicated social phobia have only a 1 in 5 chance of receiving medication. In those with comorbid depression the chance is almost 3 in 4. Long-term pharmacotherapy is increasingly common (Davidson, 1998).

In a secondary analysis of 1993–1994 psychiatric morbidity survey data, Patel and her co-workers compared 63 people suffering from social anxiety disorder with 8501 people free from psychiatric morbidity (Patel et al, 2001). The 63 social phobic cases were divided into 36 uncomplicated cases and 27 with comorbidity. People with social phobia were less likely to be in the highest socioeconomic group; they had lower employment rates and household income than those with no psychiatric morbidity, and drug dependency ran at a higher level, as did use of prescribed oral medications. Overall, there were no differences in total annual health-care costs, which averaged UK£609 in those with social phobia and £379 in the psychiatrically well population. Within the social phobia group, the costs for patients with social phobia and some comorbidity were £572 per annum compared with only £452 per annum for those with uncomplicated social phobia. The main reason for these differences was the cost of contacts with the general practitioner. These costs were much higher in cases of social phobia with comorbidity than in uncomplicated cases and the latter costs were somewhat higher than those in the psychiatrically well population. Home visits were particularly frequent in patients with complicated social phobia. In terms of employment costs there were no differences in the cost of days off work. However, there was a significantly higher value of social security benefits in the social anxiety disorder group than in the psychiatrically well population. Again, this was particularly marked in the patients with comorbidity.

Obsessive compulsive disorder

Obsessive compulsive disorder (OCD) sits uneasily among the anxiety disorders, but no better place has been found for it (Hollander et al, 1996). It has elements of anxiety, but these are not usually major. It has a lifetime prevalence of 3–5% (Pigott, 1999). One study estimated the total costs of this disorder to the US economy in 1990 at US$8 billion, 18% of the total for anxiety disorders ($46 billion). The cost of drugs in this study was $53 million, compared with $1167 million for all anxiety disorders (4.5%). Conversely, OCD patients received disproportionately expensive

hospital and medical care (Dupont et al, 1995). Obsessive compulsive disorder causes patients immense suffering, seriously jeopardizing their quality of life (Stein et al, 1996). Treatment comprises behavioural measures and/or an antidepressant acting on the serotonin-mediated pathways, such as clomipramine or the selective serotonin reuptake inhibitors (SSRIs) (Rasmussen et al, 1993).

Knapp and his associates have reviewed the cost of obsessive compulsive disorder (Knapp et al, 2000). They point out the incomplete evidence with respect to this disorder but note that it manifestly has 'quite large and wide-ranging costs'. They also note that the available evidence is mainly from the USA. To correct this, they themselves made a secondary analysis of nationally representative survey data collected in the 1984–1985 survey (Knapp et al, 2000). The rates of employment were similar between the OCD groups and the psychiatrically well population, but were significantly lower in patients with OCD with comorbidity. More OCD patients had taken time off work in the preceding year because of ill health compared with the psychiatrically well group. Again, the comorbid group had the greatest absenteeism. This group also had higher rates of service utilization including hospitalization, home visits, and counselling or therapy. No differences in medication use were apparent between the OCD group and the psychiatrically well participants, but a higher proportion of the comorbid group used psychotropic medication. A particular cost associated with the comorbid group was that of in-patient services—UK£1066 per annum, compared with only £69 in the OCD group and £346 in the well population. The cost of lost employment was four times higher in the OCD with comorbidity group and the OCD-only group but this did not quite reach significant levels. Welfare benefits were higher in the comorbid group than in the OCD-only group and the well population.

Post-traumatic stress disorder

Post-traumatic stress disorder (PTSD) is a severe condition with a lifetime prevalence of about 12.5% in women and 6.2% in men (Pigott, 1999). About one in four individuals exposed to trauma develop the syndrome. Drug treatments are still being developed, mostly using antidepressants. Few systematic data are available on the pharmacoeconomics of the condition.

Knapp's group have collaborated with the Centre for Human Sciences of the Defence Evaluation and Research Agency to evaluate the health economic considerations of PTSD (McCrone et al, in press). They have found that many factors need to be taken into account such as the prevention of PTSD, the discharge from the armed forces for military-related PTSD, and various treatment options. As yet, there are no clear estimates of the costs of treatment.

Conclusion

The anxiety disorders are common and surprisingly disabling conditions. Studies on the health economics of generalized anxiety disorder, panic disorder, social anxiety disorders and obsessive compulsive disorder document the cost to the individual and to society. Attention has focused on the 'major' psychiatric disorders such as depression, schizophrenia and the dementias. Studies suggest that many anxiety disorders are of early onset and too often chronic; they are quite common and impose a heavy burden on society. More studies will be needed to discern the fine grain in the survey material and to identify more precisely the location and type of societal costs. These factors will vary from country to country, from district to district, between men and women and between various age groups.

The pharmacoeconomics of the anxiety disorders has received little attention. In the past drug costs were largely incurred by use of benzodiazepines, most of which are available in generic forms and are cheap. They are effective and acceptable in the short term. Long-term use is associated with the risk of physical dependence, with an adverse risk–benefit ratio and high cost terms to facilitate withdrawal. There is now a trend towards the use of antidepressants in the anxiety disorders. Clinical experience has been followed by formal trial evaluation, culminating in the licensing of several SSRIs for panic and OCD (e.g. Corby and Dunne, 1997) and venlafaxine in GAD (Preskorn, 1997). The tricyclic antidepressant drugs (except imipramine and clomipramine) were not extensively used in the anxiety disorders, but the relative merits of tricyclic antidepressants and the SSRIs have been extensively debated in the indication of depression (Lane et al, 1995). The cost-effectiveness of the SSRIs has become a hotly argued issue (Woods and Baker, 1997). Overall, the consensus seems to be that SSRIs are equi-effective with tricyclic antidepressants, somewhat better tolerated, but substantially more expensive. The longer the treatment continues the less cost-effective the SSRI becomes, and long-term treatment in depression is now increasingly urged (Sechter and Lane, 1997).

Tricyclic antidepressants are not licensed for use in the anxiety disorders, so in theory the SSRIs should not be compared with them in cost-effectiveness terms. The SSRIs and venlafaxine are supplanting benzodiazepines as the latter's long-term problems become more appreciated. The SSRIs will take an increasing proportion of the market. However, in comparison with the overall costs of the anxiety disorders, this drug expenditure can be justified. Further cost-offset and cost-effectiveness studies will help hammer this point home.

One feature stands out from the studies by Knapp and his colleagues. Uncomplicated anxiety disorders do not carry much symptomatic or economic burden; however, a substantial proportion of the anxiety disorders are comorbid with other conditions such as depression and alcohol or substance misuse. In these instances economic costs multiply quite substantially. It is therefore important that in all studies a clear distinction is made between patients with uncomplicated anxiety disorders and those with comorbid conditions.

In the wider medicopolitical arena, the health cost of the anxiety disorders more than justifies pleas to accord their treatment greater prominence in health policy and research funding (Rupp et al, 1998).

References

Ballenger JC, Davidson JRT, Lecrubier Y, et al (1998). Consensus statement on Social Anxiety Disorder from the International Consensus Group on Depression and Anxiety. *J Clin Psychiatry* **59** (suppl. 17), 54–60.

Corby CL, Dunne G (1997). Paroxetine: a review. *J Serotonin Res* **4**, 47–64.

Davidson JRT (1998). Pharmacotherapy of social anxiety disorder. *J Clin Psychiatry* **59**(suppl.17), 47–51.

Dupont RL, Rice DP, Shiraki S, et al (1995). Economic costs of obsessive-compulsive disorder. *Med Interface* **89**, 102–9.

Edlund MJ, Swann AC (1987). The economic and social costs of panic disorder. *Hosp Community Psychiatry* **38**, 1277–9.

Ginsberg G, Marks I, Waters H (1984). Cost-benefit analysis of a controlled trial of nurse therapy for neurosis in primary care. *Psychol Med* 14, 683–90.

Gould RA, Otto MW, Pollack MH (1995). A meta-analysis of treatment outcome for Panic Disorder. *Clin Psychol Rev* 15, 819–44.

Greenberg PE, Sisitsky T, Kessler RC, et al (1999) The economic burden of anxiety disorders in the 1990s. *J Clin Psychiatry* 60, 427–35.

Hollander E, Kwon JH, Stein DJ, et al (1996). Obsessive-compulsive and spectrum disorders: overview and quality of life issues. *J Clin Psychiatry* 57 (suppl. 8), 3–6.

Katon W (1996). Panic disorder: relationship to high medical utilization, unexplained physical symptoms, and medical costs. *J Clin Psychiatry* 57 (suppl. 10), 11–18.

Kessler RC, McGonagle KA, Shanyang Z, et al (1994). Lifetime and 12-month prevalence of DSM-III-R psychiatric disorders in the United States. *Arch Gen Psychiatry* 51, 8–19.

Knapp M, Henderson J, Patel A (2000). Costs of obsessive-compulsive disorder: a review. In Maj M, Sartorius N, Okasha A, Zohar J, eds, *Obsessive Compulsive Disorder*. Chichester: John Wiley, 253–75.

Lane R, Baldwin D, Preskorn S (1995). The SSRIs: advantages, disadvantages and differences. *J Psychopharmacol* 9 (suppl. 2), 163–78.

Lecrubier Y (1998). Comorbidity in social anxiety disorder: impact on disease burden and management. *J Clin Psychiatry* 59 (suppl. 17), 33–7.

Leon AC, Portera L, Weissman MM (1995). The social costs of anxiety disorders. *Br J Psychiatry* 166 (suppl. 27), 19–22.

Lloyd K, Jenkins R (1995). The economics of depression in primary care. Department of Health initiatives. *Br J Psychiatry* 166 (suppl. 27), 60–2.

Lowman RL (1991). Mental health claims experience: analysis and benefit redesign. *Prof Psychol Res Pract* 22, 36–44.

McCrone P, Knapp M, Cawkill P (2001). Post-traumatic stress disorder (PTSD) in the UK Armed Forces: health economic consideration. In press.

McCusker J, Boulenger JP, Boyer R et al (1997). Use of health services for anxiety disorders: a multisite study in Quebec. *Can J Psychiatry* 42, 730–6.

Narrow WE, Regier DA, Rae DS, et al (1993). Use of services by persons with mental and addictive disorders. Findings from the National Institute of Mental Health Epidemiologic Catchment Area Program. *Arch Gen Psychiatry* 50, 95–107.

Nutt D, Baldwin D, Beaumont G, et al (1999). Guidelines for the management of social phobia/social anxiety disorder. *Primary Care Psychiatry* 5, 147–55.

Patel A, Knapp M, Henderson J, Baldwin D (2001). The economic consequences of social phobia. *J Affect Disord* Forthcoming.

Pigott TA (1999). Gender differences in the epidemiology and treatment of anxiety disorders. *J Clin Psychiatry* 60 (suppl. 18), 4–15.

Preskorn A (1997). Pharmacotherapeutic profile of venlafaxine. *Eur Psychiatry* 12 (suppl. 4), 285–94s.

Rasmussen SA, Eisen JL, Pato MT (1993). Current issues in the pharmacologic management of obsessive compulsive disorder. *J Clin Psychiatry* 54 (suppl. 6), 4–9.

Rees CS, Richards JC, Smith LM (1998). Medical utilisation and costs in panic disorder: a comparison with social phobia. *J Anxiety Disord* 12, 421–35.

Rice DP, Miller LS (1995). The economic burden of affective disorders. *Br J Psychiatry* **166** (suppl. 27), 34–42.

Rice DP, Miller LS (1998). Health economics and cost implications of anxiety and other mental disorders in the United States. *Br J Psychiatry* **173** (suppl. 34), 4–9.

Roy-Byrne PP (1996). Generalized anxiety and mixed anxiety-depression: association with disability and health care utilization. *J Clin Psychiatry* **57** (suppl. 7), 86–91.

Rupp A, Gause EM, Regier, DA (1998). Research policy implications of cost-of-illness studies for mental disorders. *Br J Psychiatry* **173** (suppl. 36), 19–25.

Salvador-Carulla L, Segui J, Fernandez-Cano P, et al (1995). Costs and offset effect in panic disorders. *Br J Psychiatry* **166** (suppl. 27), 23–8.

Sechter D, Lane RM (1997). Continuation therapy with selective serotonin re-uptake inhibitors. *J Serotonin Res* **4**, 65–111.

Shah A, Jenkins R (2000). Mental health economic studies from developing countries reviewed in the context of those from developed countries. *Acta Psychiatr Scand* **101**, 87–103.

Simon G, Ormel J, VonKorff M, et al (1995). Health care costs associated with depressive and anxiety disorders in primary care. *Am J Psychiatry* **152**, 352–7.

Souetre E, Lozet H, Cimarosti I, et al (1994). Cost of anxiety disorders: impact of comorbidity. *J Psychosom Res* **38** (suppl. 1), 151–60.

Stein DJ, Roberts M, Hollander E, et al (1996). Quality of life and pharmaco-economic aspects of obsessive-compulsive disorder. A South African survey. *S Afr Med J* **86**, 1579–85.

Woods SW, Baker CB (1997). Cost-effectiveness of newer antidepressants. *Curr Opin Psychiatry* **10**, 95–101.

World Health Organization (1992). *The ICD-10 Classification.* Geneva: WHO.

Zaubler TS, Katon K (1998). Panic disorder in the general medical setting. *J Psychosom Res* **44**, 5–42.

Bipolar affective disorder

John Cookson

5

Bipolar disorder, previously known as manic–depressive disorder, is a mental illness characterized by severe mood swings in the direction of either depression or exaggerated feelings of well-being accompanied by a syndrome of other symptoms (mania) (Goodwin and Jamison, 1990). These episodes have a recurring pattern but generally subside spontaneously after a period of weeks or months. Between episodes the patient is relatively free of symptoms, with a restoration of normal function. What distinguishes bipolar disorder from other affective disorders, such as recurrent depression, is a history of mania or hypomania (a milder form). As well as elation and irritability of mood, the syndrome of mania includes increased energy, decreased need for sleep, overactivity mostly of a purposeful kind, grandiosity which may become delusional, disinhibition or indiscreet behaviour, a speeding-up of thought processes manifest in pressure of speech and flight of ideas, and distractibility, attention easily being drawn away by chance sights and sounds. Mania is a particularly insightless illness.

Depression often follows a manic episode (bipolar I disorder), but in other cases the main disorder presents as depressive episodes which are followed by or sometimes preceded by hypomanic swings (bipolar II disorder).

Bipolar disorder usually begins in early adulthood and affects approximately 1% of the population. The cause of the disorder is largely unknown although hereditary factors play an important part, and major life events often precede the onset of the first episode of the disorder, and less obviously subsequent episodes.

Although the diagnostic criteria for mania are described consistently in all the major diagnostic systems, it is common to find that a patient with diagnosed bipolar disorder has at earlier stages in life been diagnosed, probably incorrectly, as having a variety of other disorders, ranging from schizophrenia to personality disorder. The diagnosis is also complicated by comorbidity with other conditions, particularly substance misuse.

Depression occurring as part of bipolar disorder may be severe and accompanied by ideas of guilt and hopelessness, an inability to function at work because of poor concentration and psychomotor retardation or agitation, poor judgement and suicidal ideation. The lifelong risk of suicide in people with this condition is as high as 15%. Factors associated with suicide risk include alcohol misuse, marital separation or divorce, living alone and unemployment, and these are all common secondary consequences of the illness.

There is great variety in the frequency and severity of episodes from one individual to another with this diagnosis. A few patients enter a phase of rapid cycling in which they have four or more episodes a year. There is also variety in the qualitative presentation of symptoms. Some patients tend to have more elated and grandiose patterns of mania, while others present as irritable, hostile and suspicious; the latter are more likely to infringe the law and to come to medical attention through the courts or prison system. Although both the manic and depressive episodes are usually self-terminating, lasting damage can result from the social consequences, particularly during a manic episode. Thus patients may behave in a disrespectful, irresponsible or outrageous way at work or at home, and may find it difficult to achieve a return to their former status at work or to sustain their marriage.

Treatment

Drug treatment is a vital part of the management of bipolar disorder, both during episodes of depression or mania and as prophylaxis thereafter. Patients require explanation and education about the illness and about the treatments available, in order to be able to make informed choices and to avail themselves of the appropriate options for treatment.

The treatments for depression are similar to those for other types of depressive illness.

There is, however, a unique risk in the bipolar form that antidepressant treatment may trigger a switch into mania. This may occur either as the natural outcome of recovery from depression or as a pharmacological effect of the drug. Particular antidepressants (the selective serotonin reuptake inhibitors) seem less liable to induce the switch into mania than other antidepressants or electroconvulsive therapy. Treatment for mania consists initially of antipsychotic medication, for instance the widely used haloperidol, often combined with other less specific sedative medication such as the benzodiazepines (lorazepam intramuscularly or diazepam orally). The manic state will usually begin to subside within hours and this improvement develops further over the next 2 weeks. If the patient remains disturbed with manic symptoms, additional treatment with a 'mood stabilizer' may help.

The first mood stabilizer was lithium (its antimanic action being discovered in 1948); more recently the anticonvulsant drugs carbamazepine and valproate have been found to be effective in acute mania. Unfortunately these mood stabilizers are only successful in controlling mania to a limited extent and few patients are well enough to leave hospital at the end of 3 weeks of treatment using these drugs as monotherapy. It is increasingly common for combination treatment to be advocated, in which an antipsychotic drug is combined with lithium or an anticonvulsant, or with both lithium and valproate. American authors and the guidelines of the American Psychiatric Association (1994) advocate the avoidance of antipsychotic drugs in bipolar disorder because they fear the development of tardive dyskinesia. This is a pattern of abnormal involuntary movements affecting especially the mouth, tongue and face, and occurring during long-term treatment with antipsychotic drugs. Despite this advice, the majority of patients with acute mania in Europe and in the USA are treated with antipsychotic drugs in combination with others and remain on these drugs at the time of discharge from hospital and even 6 months later (Cookson and Sachs, 1999). New atypical antipsychotic agents cause fewer extrapyramidal side effects, and there is preliminary evidence of a lower risk of tardive dyskinesia during long-term treatment with certain of these drugs. The atypical drugs that have been shown in placebo-controlled trials to be effective either alone or in combination with lithium or valproate in mania are olanzapine and risperidone.

The 'mood stabilizers' were so called because they prevent recurrences of mood swings in people with bipolar disorder. The evidence for this is best with lithium, but is based on studies carried out more than 20 years ago. However, recent naturalistic surveys tend to find that lithium is far less useful in general clinical practice than in research settings. Many patients discontinue lithium within less than a year, giving as their reasons side effects and doubt about their need for treatment. A survey by Johnson and McFarland (1996) estimated the total number of days of lithium treatment after initiation of prescription. The patients were involved in a 6-year longitudinal cohort study in an American insurance scheme. Patients who were prescribed lithium took it for only 38% of the time they were enrolled in the plan. Only 9% of patients used lithium for 90% of the time enrolled. They had an average of 1.4 mental health visits per month of lithium use. Discontinuation of lithium was associated with hospitalization for psychiatric problems. In even the best-run specialist lithium clinics only some 23% of patients commenced on lithium derive a very good outcome over 5 years, which is freedom from a further severe episode that would usually require hospitalization (Maj et al, 1998).

In the case of carbamazepine the evidence suggests that its prophylactic efficacy is less than that of lithium (Greil and Kleindienst, 1999). For valproate there is no placebo-controlled evidence as yet to support its efficacy in the prophylaxis of bipolar disorder. The only large-scale study designed to elucidate this action was a failed trial in which neither lithium nor valproate was more effective than placebo in maintenance treatment over 2 years (Bowden et al, 2000).

Side effects

Lithium can cause tremor, weight gain and mental dulling as well as endocrine abnormalities affecting the thyroid gland and urinary flow. Of particular importance is the toxicity of lithium in concentrations only slightly higher than those required for therapeutic effects. Lithium toxicity is associated with acute gastrointestinal disturbance such as vomiting and diarrhoea, together with drowsiness, confusion and even coma, and neurological symptoms resulting from cerebellar dysfunction. If the toxicity lasts for more than a few days it is liable to cause permanent neurological damage with cerebellar impairment, resulting in the patient being unable to walk and having extremely slurred speech. Such episodes of toxicity can result from the inadvertent combination of other drugs (e.g. thiazide diuretics, non-steroidal anti-inflammatory drugs or certain antibiotics) with lithium, or through the occurrence of an intercurrent physical illness such as pneumonia. Patients taking lithium require regular blood tests to measure lithium levels, and to check thyroid and renal function every year. The blood tests should be carried out more frequently if there is any instability in the patient's physical or mental health or any change in medication. Patients need to be educated on a continuing basis about their illness and treatment.

Carbamazepine is associated with acute

nausea if the dose is increased too quickly, and with ataxia. A more serious side effect of carbamazepine is an allergic reaction resulting most commonly in a rash (occurring in up to 15% of patients) and rarely in agranulocytosis or the Stevens–Johnson syndrome with inflammation of mucous membranes including pneumonitis and oesophagitis. The latter is fatal if not dealt with urgently. Blood counts are advisable in patients on carbamazepine 2–4 weeks after starting treatment.

Valproate is generally tolerated better than lithium or carbamazepine but can cause long-term weight gain. In younger people it has been associated with acute liver damage. It is not generally necessary to monitor blood levels of either carbamazepine or valproate, although such tests can aid in checking compliance and sometimes in arriving at the right therapeutic dose.

Quality of life

The symptoms of bipolar disorder and the side effects associated with its treatment have implications for the patient's health-related quality of life. The disorder itself has an impact upon mental and emotional well-being. Bipolar disorder also affects areas of life such as employment, social partnerships and independence. The side effects of treatment may further impair the quality of life. Treatment with lithium can reduce the risk of suicide (Muller-Oerlinghausen and Berghofer, 1999).

Economic impact of bipolar disorder

Bipolar disorder has an economic impact on the patient, on those who pay for health care, and on society as a whole. The patients' erratic behaviour may impair their ability to make financial decisions. Their functioning at work may deteriorate, compromising their ability to maintain a stable income, through absence from work and low productivity during periods of illness. Relapses often require intensive psychiatric attention including hospitalization or community support to restore the patient's behaviour towards normal, to protect other people and to prevent suicide. Drug therapy, although a factor, is a relatively small part of the total cost of the condition compared with the provision of emergency services for acute mania or depression. Indirect costs arise from the loss of productivity of the patients and their caregivers.

Health economic studies of bipolar disorder and its treatment

The sources of direct costs include the costs of hospitalization in psychiatric hospitals or general medical wards, and the costs of medication and laboratory tests. Out-patient costs may include occasional reviews by a psychiatrist, general practice attendance, and for some patients additional input from a clinical psychologist or community psychiatric nurse. In more severe cases there may be costs for social benefits including supported accommodation. The direct costs and secondary consequences of the disorder include those arising from criminal infringements including incarceration in prison, and those associated with the misuse of alcohol and drugs.

Indirect costs are related mainly to employment, in particular reduced levels of productivity at work, and absence due to sickness, as well as the mortality of the disease. Caregiving by the family is an opportunity cost associated with the illness.

Crucial factors affecting overall cost are the responsiveness to medication (for example, less than 70% of patients are 'lithium responders'), adherence to recommended treatment, and adverse events resulting from medication. A particular hazard of lithium treatment is the risk of rapid re-emergence of mania, which occurs in up to 50% of patients if the drug is abruptly discontinued (see Cookson, 1997). Disappointingly, it has not been found that the introduction of widespread treatment with lithium has been associated with a reduction in the number of patients admitted and discharged from hospital with a diagnosis of mania. In order to achieve the best result with the available

treatments, it may be necessary to have specialist affective disorders clinics ('lithium clinics') in order to optimize the delivery of treatment.

Studies of the cost of treatment of individual patients for a year show a range from US$3254 (Bauer et al, 1997) to $50 856 (Keck et al, 1996a). Costs vary depending upon characteristics of the illness, such as frequency of cycling of episodes, and the presence of mixed as opposed to the classical elated mania. In general, patients with mixed affective states were found to carry the highest costs, those with rapid cycling disorder slightly lower costs, and those with classical symptoms the lowest: $31 426 for 1 year (Keck et al, 1996).

Sajatovic et al (1997) performed a retrospective 2-year study examining differences in health resource utilization associated with different drug treatments for acute mania. They found no statistically significant difference between the groups. The patients on multiple mood stabilizers were more likely to have comorbid psychiatric conditions and their mean length of stay in hospital was 30 days compared with patients on lithium (21 days) and on anticonvulsants (17 days). Likewise, Bauer et al (1997) found the mean length of stay in hospital ranged from 13 days to 35 days depending on the type of mania and the drugs used. This was a prospective study on resource utilization by 103 bipolar patients over 1 year in a Veterans Affairs clinic.

The total cost of illness includes direct and indirect costs. This has been calculated as ranging from US$30 billion to $45 billion annually in the USA in the period 1990–93 (Greenberg et al, 1993; Wyatt and Henter, 1995; Rice and Miller, 1995). The total loss of earnings due to mortality (suicide) ranged from $6 billion to $7.5 billion. The total earnings lost through reduced productivity and absence from work ranged from $1 billion to $26 billion.

The total costs are likely to reflect the efficacy of treatment. In one industry-sponsored study (Keck et al, 1996b) treatment with lithium or valproate was compared in relation to classical, mixed and rapid-cycling disorder. Treatment with lithium was associated with lower costs than treatment with valproate for classical bipolar disorder, but treatment with valproate was associated with lower costs than treatment with lithium for mixed and rapid-cycling disorders. This is in keeping with the evidence that valproate is more effective than lithium for certain patients with rapid-cycling disorder and probably also for certain patients with mixed affective states. However, these associations are a guide to predicting response to treatment but are not very specific.

US/UK differences

Studies of health economics in the UK and the USA in unipolar depressive illness show substantial differences, with for example estimates of total costs of $0.8 billion in the UK, and $44 billion in the USA where the population is about five times larger (Greenberg et al, 1993; Kind and Sorensen, 1993). Likewise, in a study of the costs of bipolar disorder in the UK (Das Gupta et al, 2001), the direct health-care costs were estimated to be about UK£285 million, compared with the equivalent of UK£3 billion in the USA (Wyatt and Henter, 1995). In particular, after adjusting for population sizes, annual in-patient costs were estimated as being six times higher in the USA. Total costs were £2 billion, compared with the figures of $30–45 billion in the USA (see above).

Discussion

Few papers have looked at the economic implications of bipolar affective disorder. Most of the published studies look at direct medical costs over the course of a year. Industry-sponsored studies focus on the benefits of a new treatment over older treatments. However, factors individual to a particular patient are likely to be more important than the average cost of a particular treatment. These include selection of patients who are likely to respond to a particular treatment, and psychoeducation coupled with encouragement during follow-up and careful monitoring, to avoid such expensive outcomes as full-blown relapse, serious toxicity or suicide.

Acknowledgement

I am grateful to Inge Duchesne for assistance in researching articles for this manuscript.

References

American Psychiatric Association (1994). Practice guideline for the treatment of patients with bipolar disorder. *Am J Psychiatry* **151** (suppl. 12), 1–36.

Bauer MS, Shea N, McBride L, Gavin C (1997). Predictors of service utilization in veterans with bipolar disorder: a prospective study. *J Affective Disord* **44**, 159–68.

Bowden CL, Calabrese JR, McElroy SL, et al (2000). A randomised, placebo-controlled 12-month trial of divalproex and lithium in treatment of outpatients with bipolar I disorder. *Arch Gen Psychiatry* **57**, 481–9.

Cookson JC (1997). Lithium: balancing risks and benefits. *Br J Psychiatry* **171**, 120–4.

Cookson JC, Sachs GS (1999). Lithium: clinical use in mania and prophylaxis of affective disorders. In: Buckley PF, Waddington JL, eds, *Schizophrenia and Mood Disorders: The New Drug Therapies in Clinical Practice.* Oxford: Butterworth Heinemann.

Das Gupta R, Wright T, Guest JF (2001). The annual cost of bipolar disorder to UK society. *Int J Psychiatry.*

Goodwin FK, Jamison KR (1990). *Manic-Depressive Illness.* Oxford: Oxford University Press.

Greenberg PE, Stiglin LE, Finkelstein SN, Berndt ER (1993). The economic burden of depression in 1990. *J Clin Psychiatry* **54**, 405–18.

Greil W, Kleindienst N (1999). The comparative prophylactic efficacy of lithium and carbamazepine in patients with bipolar I disorder. *Int Clin Psychopharmacol* **14**, 277–81.

Johnson RE, McFarland BH (1996). Lithium use and discontinuation in a health maintenance organisation. *Am J Psychiatry* **153**, 993–1000.

Keck PE, McElroy SL, Bennett JA (1996a). Health-economic implications of the onset of action of antimanic agents. *J Clin Psychiatry* **57** (suppl. 13), 13–18.

Keck PE, Nabulsi AA, Taylor JL, et al (1996b). A pharmacoeconomic model of divalproex vs. lithium in the acute and prophylactic treatment of bipolar I disorder. *J Clin Psychiatry* **57**, 213–22.

Kind P, Sorensen J (1993). The cost of depression. *Int Clin Psychopharmacol* **7**, 191–5.

Maj M, Pirozzi R, Magliano L, et al (1998). Long-term outcome of lithium prophylaxis in bipolar disorder 5-year prospective study of 402 patients a lithium clinic. *Am J Psychiatry* **155**, 30–5.

Muller-Oerlinghausen B, Berghofer A (1999). Antidepressants and suicide risk. *J Clin Psychiatry* **60** (suppl. 2), 94–9.

Rice DP, Miller LS (1995). The economic burden of affective disorders. *Br J Psychiatry* **166** (suppl. 27), 34–42.

Sajatovic M, Gerhart C, Semple W (1997). Association between mood-stabilizing medication and mental health resource use in the management of acute mania. *Psychiatr Serv* **48**, 1037–41.

Wyatt RJ, Henter I (1995). An economic evaluation of manic-depressive illness—1991. *Soc Psychiatry Psychiatr Epidemiol* **30**, 213–19.

Dementia: evidence and issues

Linda M Davies and Andrea Manca

6

People with dementia and their carers require access to a variety of health and social care services for treatment, information and counselling, community-based support, respite care and long-term residential care. Treatment may include behavioural therapies (e.g. reality orientation, cognitive stimulation and validation therapy) or pharmacological treatment with acetylcholinesterase inhibitors.

Dementia imposes substantial medical, social, psychological and financial costs on patients, their families and friends, as well as on health and social services. The progressive nature of the illness and the ageing of the population mean that many people with dementia will require intensive support and/or long-term residential or nursing home care.

The costs of care for people with cognitive disability in the UK have been estimated at between UK £14 926 and £47 232 per person (updated to 1997/8 costs), depending on the severity of disability and the setting of care (Kavanagh et al, 1993; Kavanagh and Knapp, 1999). Reports of the total costs of care for people with dementia in the UK range from £1 billion to £6 billion per year (Gray and Fenn, 1993; Bosanquet et al, 1998; Manca and Davies, 1999). These estimates suggest that between 2% and 13% of the total health and personal social services expenditure is for the care of people with dementia or Alzheimer's disease.

Concerns about the high cost of health and social care are compounded by the introduction of pharmaceutical products such as the acetylcholinesterase inhibitors. Currently, these drugs are considered to be the most successful agents for the management of dementia, primarily Alzheimer's disease (Burns et al, 1999). Second-generation cholinesterase inhibitors (e.g. donepezil, rivastigmine) have been reported to have similar efficacy and safety results, in terms of improved cognitive function and delayed progression of disease in some patients. The National Institute for Clinical Excellence (NICE) has recommended that three drugs should be made available on the National Health Service for people with mild to moderate Alzheimer's disease and Mini-Mental State Examination scores of 12 points or more (NICE, 2001). However, NICE also recognizes that there is significant uncertainty about the costs of the drugs and associated health and social care. This is compounded by the fact that the value of the drugs to patients and carers in terms of improved quality of life is unclear (NICE, 2001).

At a time of rising expenditure and budget constraints, all health-care systems require evidence about the value for money of the care provided. This includes comparisons of the relative costs and patient benefits for different diseases, and comparisons of alternative therapeutic strategies for each specific disease.

Institutionalization has been identified as one of the main cost drivers in the care of people with dementia (Holmes et al, 1998; Souêtre et al, 1999), and the savings achieved by delaying the onset of institutionalization for these patients are expected to offset the additional drug acquisition costs.

A number of economic studies have been published that assess the economic impact of the introduction of anticholinesterase drugs on the care for people with dementia. Overall, they suggest that the introduction of the new drugs might be cost-neutral, while leading to modest improvements in the health-related quality of life of patients and carers. However, the reliability and robustness of the economic evidence need to be considered before concluding that any additional benefits of the new drugs for dementia are indeed worth the cost.

Methods of pharmacoeconomics

The objective of economic evaluations of health and social care interventions is to inform decision-makers about the relative costs and benefits to society of two or more methods of providing care. In the context of dementia these may be comparisons of different drug therapies (pharmacoeconomic evaluations), or comparisons of behavioural interventions or packages of care. To achieve this aim, any economic evaluation must be based on a broad perspective which includes the costs of all resources or services used as inputs to the process of providing care and the benefits to society of the outcome of care. For people with dementia, the costs are likely to include health care provided by primary and secondary care services such as general practitioner visits, hospital in-patient and out-patient services for assessment and follow-up, social care services such as residential accommodation and support of carers, and the value of time spent by informal carers such as family or friends. The benefits are improvements in the health of patients and informal carers due to increased survival and/or health-related quality of life.

There are four types of economic evaluation: cost-minimization analysis, cost-effectiveness analysis, cost-utility analysis and cost-benefit analysis. The analytic framework chosen will depend upon the economic questions posed and the clinical evidence of effectiveness for the interventions (Gold et al, 1996; Drummond et al, 1997).

Cost-minimization analysis

Cost-minimization analysis compares the direct costs of two or more health-care interventions. This form of analysis is only useful if there is clear and reliable evidence that there is no difference in patient outcomes between two or more interventions.

Cost-effectiveness analysis

Cost-effectiveness analysis uses measures of clinical effectiveness to quantify the benefits of care. For dementia, measures such as years of life with mild or moderate disability, or change in cognitive function, are used. If one intervention—such as a new drug to control symptoms or delay progression—leads to lower direct costs and improved patient outcomes, it is dominant and the preferred option. That is, it clearly saves resources to provide care and is more beneficial to the patient. More often, a new therapy is associated with improved patient outcomes at additional cost. Incremental cost-effectiveness ratios (ICER) provide a measure of the cost of gaining a unit of health improvement, such as cost per year of life gained. The ICER is calculated as (cost of A − cost of B)/(outcome of A − outcome of B). The use of a single measure of effectiveness in the denominator means that cost-effectiveness analysis may be of limited value in situations where a range of outcomes are important (such as the impact of an intervention and associated adverse events on survival and on physical, social and emotional function).

Cost-utility analysis

Cost-utility analysis is similar to cost-effectiveness analysis in approach, but uses utility as the outcome measure. The utility value is a measure that combines preferences for and values of the overall effect of an intervention on survival, physical and mental health, and social function. Utility is combined with estimates of length of life to provide an assessment of quality-adjusted life years (QALYs). As in cost-effectiveness analysis, incremental cost-utility ratios are calculated to estimate the cost of producing one extra QALY.

Cost-benefit analysis

Cost-benefit analysis uses monetary valuations of the morbidity and mortality consequences of diseases or interventions. This allows estimation of the absolute and relative net social benefit of intervention, calculated as the monetary value of the consequences of an intervention minus the direct costs. Any health or social care intervention with a net social benefit greater than zero (i.e. the benefits are greater than the costs) is worth undertaking. Two approaches have typically been used to value outcomes in monetary values. The first is the human capital approach, where the monetary value of benefit represents the value of changes in the amount or type of work done or use of leisure time as

a consequence of morbidity or mortality. They are also called productivity or time costs (Gold et al, 1996; Drummond et al, 1997). However, these do not incorporate valuation of preferences for length of life or health and social well-being.

The second approach estimates the monetary value to individuals and society of health and social well-being and life *per se*. In practical terms this requires assessment of the amount of money which individuals would accept as compensation for reductions in health or life expectancy, or the amount they would be prepared to pay for improvements in health or life expectancy. The methodology for this approach is still being tested and developed.

Review of the evidence

A systematic search of published literature identified 13 studies concerned with the value for money of acetylcholinesterase inhibitors. The majority were cost analyses of the potential savings in providing health and social care which may accrue from the introduction of these drugs. However, the available clinical evidence is not sufficient to support the assumption that acetylcholinesterase inhibitors are equivalent to other interventions in terms of clinical effect or side effects (Birks and Melzer, 1999; NICE, 2001). Furthermore, research to assess potential cost savings implicitly assumes that the drugs may be superior in terms of clinical effectiveness. These factors indicate that a cost analysis is not an appropriate framework for the economic evaluation of the new drugs.

Four studies formally compared both costs and outcomes. These were cost-effectiveness analyses of donepezil, in the UK (Stewart et al, 1998), Canada (O'Brien et al, 1998), the USA (Neumann et al, 1999), and Sweden (Jönsson et al, 1999b). Table 6.1 summarizes their results. To compare across the different settings, the costs have been converted to a single currency (US dollars) using a Health Purchasing Power Parity price index (OECD, 1999). This adjusts for some of the structural differences in the organization and costs of health services between countries. Overall, the studies indicate that donepezil is associated with a net improvement in the 'number of years spent in a non-severe condition' of between 1 month and 6 months. The net costs of donepezil were similarly varied, ranging from a saving of US$1962 to an additional cost of US$1333. All of the authors noted that these results are preliminary and uncertain. To inform health and social care providers and policy-makers about the potential impact of new interventions in practice, a number of issues need to be considered when interpreting the available evidence.

Perspective of analysis

Economic studies should consider the costs of all the resources and services used in the process of care. In addition, the outcomes that are a consequence of the health or social care interventions evaluated need to be included. For dementia, these include the costs of hospital in-patient and out-patient care, primary and community-based health-care services, social welfare services, and care provided by voluntary agencies or by family and friends. Ideally, a broad perspective reflecting the costs and outcomes to society should be adopted. As a minimum, the perspective of the analysis should include the costs and outcomes to key health and social care providers or funders and to patients and their families.

However, the perspective and range of costs included differed between the studies. Some authors included both direct costs and informal carers' time (O'Brien et al, 1998; Stewart et al, 1998; Neumann et al, 1999) whereas others only considered direct medical costs (Jönsson et al, 1999b). If the new drugs are effective in preventing progression of the disease or in relieving symptoms, this may reduce the use of formal care services, captured by the costs of medical and social care, but increase the burden on family and friends. In this situation, excluding informal care costs from the analysis may result in overestimation of the relative cost-effectiveness of the new drugs.

Table 6.1
Estimated costs and benefits of donepezil for people with Alzheimer's disease.

Study	Outcome measure	Year of costing	Original currency	Incremental cost[a] (US$)	Incremental Outcome
Stewart et al (1998)	Expected life years in condition less than severe	1997	GB pounds	1333	0.120
O'Brien et al (1999)	Expected life years in condition less than severe	1997	Canadian dollars	−1292	0.200
Jönsson et al (1999b)	Expected life years in condition less than severe	1998	Swedish kronor	−1962	0.522
Neumann et al (1999)	Quality-adjusted life years	1997	US dollars	483	0.015

[a]Costs converted to US dollars (1996 value) using the Health Purchasing Power Parity price index (OECD, 1999).

Time frame of analysis

Economic studies should cover the full period over which the interventions could be expected to have an effect on resource use, survival and health-related quality of life. However, the economic evaluations of donepezil were based on effectiveness data from a limited number of trials, which were short in duration. This has a number of implications. First, the analysis can be limited to the effect of the drug during the period for which effectiveness data were available. In this case, it may be assumed that the treatment effect ceased after 6 months (Stewart et al, 1998). This assumption would only be valid if the donepezil were also discontinued at 6 months. If this is not the case, then the overall costs of the drug may be underestimated and the benefits overestimated.

Alternatively, some studies used expert opinion to extrapolate the effectiveness of donepezil over a longer period (Neumann et al, 1999; O'Brien et al, 1999). However, it is recognized that expert opinion can be the weakest source of evidence, which introduces considerable uncertainty into the analysis and interpretation of the results. In addition, the cost-effectiveness of acetylcholinesterase inhibitors depends heavily on the distribution of the cohort of patients across different severity states. O'Brien's team found that the results of their model were very sensitive to this variable. In this context, the correct assessment of the duration of the treatment effect of anticholinesterase drugs assumes a central role since it will affect the number of people having mild to moderate Alzheimer's disease at each period of time.

Target population and comparators

The population considered in the analysis should be representative of the population to be treated. The trial and observational data used for the economic evaluations of donepezil may not meet this criterion. The trials have been criticized (Birks and Melzer, 1999) for enrolling carefully selected subgroups of patients with mild to moderate dementia and excluding those with coexisting illness or concurrent treatment. In addition, the observational data used may not be representative of dementia or Alzheimer's disease patient populations. These two factors reduce the generalizability of the results of the economic evaluations to patient groups outside the trial setting.

The interventions compared need to be relevant to the health and social care choices faced by decision-makers. Unless 'do nothing' is a valid management strategy, comparison of a new intervention with placebo is not appropriate for an economic evaluation. Since there are a number of drug therapies and non-pharmacological approaches to the management of people with dementia, the relative cost-effectiveness of these needs to be assessed. For example, there is a lack of 'head-to-head' comparisons of the different antidementia drugs. Once it is established that antidementia drugs are cost-effective it is important to compare these drugs within the same experimental setting.

Measurement and evaluation of costs

To be useful to those concerned with choices in the allocation of health and social care resources, the data for economic evaluations need to be timely, relevant, credible and accurate (Davies, 1998). As a minimum, the costs associated with the interventions should be estimated from activity data, which quantify resources used, and price or unit cost data. Often evidence from well-controlled prospective trials with high internal validity is required to establish whether differences in economic end points are directly attributable to the interventions. However, the economic evaluations of acetylcholinesterase inhibitors estimated costs from retrospective analysis of available datasets (Jönsson et al, 1999b), analysis of published literature (e.g. Stewart et al, 1998) and expert opinion (e.g. O'Brien et al, 1999; Neumann et al, 1999). This means that it is not clear whether differences in costs were due to the anticholinesterase inhibitors or to other factors such as availability of services in different areas, the living situation of the patient, or disease severity.

Three analyses (O'Brien et al, 1999; Stewart et al, 1998; Jönsson et al, 1999a) directly or indirectly used a measure of disease severity—Mini-Mental State Examination (MMSE) scale—to explore the link between treatment costs and disease progression. The MMSE score was strongly correlated with the costs of dementia care, but the robustness of this instrument as a cost predictor is uncertain. It has been suggested (Jönsson et al, 1999a) that there might be other tools that have strong correlation with costs, such as those measuring activities of daily living and behavioural disturbances.

Measurement and evaluation of outcomes

It is crucial that an economic study includes the health-related consequences of morbidity and mortality. These could be measured as number of years of life lost, reductions in health status, and quality of remaining years of life due to morbidity for both patients and informal carers. These consequences should also be valued to reflect the preferences of individuals and society for changes in the length and quality of life or health.

Three of the four studies discussed above measured the benefits of anticholinesterase inhibitors as 'time spent in condition less than severe'. While this provides a measure of health status, it does not give an assessment of the value to patients or society of the health gained. In addition, the measure of disease severity was based on the cognitive status of the patient, which is only one dimension of the overall health-related and non-health-related quality of life. Other factors such as behavioural disturbances and general activities of daily living (such as dressing, bathing and handling finances) have a considerable impact on patients' and carers' quality of life. These factors are also likely to affect the need for and use of health and social care services and informal care. This highlights the need to ensure that the data used to evaluate and compare interventions adequately capture the interrelationship between costs and outcomes.

One study used quality-adjusted life years to capture the range of health-related dimensions that may affect the quality of life of patients. This measure also provides an estimate of the value or preferences for changes in health status (Neumann et al, 1999). The study used the Health Utility Index Mark II in a sample of patients and carers, which is a generic measure of the value of health-related quality of life. However, it is clear that further research is needed to explore (a) the key determinants or dimensions of quality of life that are important to people with dementia and their carers; (b) whether existing instruments to measure and value health-related quality of life are able to detect differences in quality of life that are important to people with cognitive disability and their carers; and (c) whether the assessment and valuations of health-related quality of life differ between people with dementia and proxy respondents. The latter may include informal carers or health and social care professionals who complete the instruments on behalf of the patient.

Conclusion

Care for people with dementia is demanding of resources, while the outcomes of care are uncertain. To date, the economic analyses of care strategies have been limited to new drug therapies for people with Alzheimer's disease. Full economic evaluations to compare both the costs and consequences have only been conducted for one of these drugs, donepezil. However, problems with the design and data used in these studies mean that they do not provide robust evidence to determine appropriate management strategies for dementia.

In the near future new drugs for the treatment of Alzheimer's disease are expected to be licensed, and it would be extremely valuable to be able to compare them in a clear and well-defined framework. In addition, if economic evaluation is to inform health and social care providers and policy-makers about the potential impact of new interventions in practice, estimation of the value for money of these new interventions requires consideration of (a) the perceived and objective risks and benefits of care; (b) attitudes of people with dementia, carers and health and social care providers to risk; (c) the utility to these groups of health-care interventions; and (d) the uncertainty surrounding estimates of risk, utility and costs.

Further primary and secondary research is required to provide robust estimates of the formal and informal care costs associated with the new drugs and the value of health improvements to patients and carers.

Search details

An electronic and manual search of the published literature was used to identify economic analyses of cholinesterase inhibitors. In addition the bibliographies of the retrieved articles were reviewed in order to identify further relevant publications. Studies were identified performing searches on Medline, EMBASE, BIDS, Cochrane Library, DH-Data, EconLit, NHS EED, King's Fund Database, HTA database and NHS DARE between 1993 and 2000, where possible. The following terms were combined: Alzheimer's disease, dementia, cognitive impairment, drug treatment, drug therapy, anti-dementia drugs, anticholinesterase drugs, cholinesterase inhibitors, cognitive disability, cost-effectiveness analysis, cost utility analysis, cost benefit analysis, resources use, economics, costs, economic evaluation.

References

Birks JS, Melzer D (1999). Donepezil for mild and moderate Alzheimer's disease (Cochrane Review). In: *The Cochrane Library*, Issue 4, Oxford: Update Software.

Bosanquet N, May J, Johnson N (1998) Alzheimer's disease in the United Kingdom. Burden of disease and future care. Health Policy Review paper 12. Health Policy Unit, Imperial College School of Medicine, London.

Burns A, Russell E, Page S (1999). New drugs for Alzheimer's disease. *Br J Psychiatry* **174**, 476–9.

Corey-Bloom J, Anand R, Veach J, for the ENA 713 B352 Study Group (1998). A randomised trial evaluating the efficacy and safety of ENA 713 (rivastigmine tartrate), a new acetylcholinesterase inhibitor, in patients with mild and moderately severe Alzheimer's disease. *Int J Geriatr Psychopharmacol* **1**, 55–65.

Davies LM (1998). Economic evaluation in clinical trials. *Appl Clin Trials* **7**, 62–70.

Drummond MF, O'Brien B, Stoddard GL, Torrance GW (1997). *Methods for the Economic Evaluation of Health Care Programmes*, 2nd edn. New York: Oxford University Press.

Fenn P, Gray A (1999). Estimating long term cost savings from treatment of Alzheimer's disease. A modelling approach. *Pharmacoeconomics* **16**, 165–74.

Gray AM, Fenn P (1993). Alzheimer's disease: the burden of illness in England. *Health Trends* **25**, 31–7.

Gold MR, Siegel JE, Russel LB, Weinstein MG (1996). Cost-Effectiveness in Health and Medicine. New York: Oxford University Press.

Holmes J, Pugner K, Phillips R, Dempsey G, Cayton H (1998). Managing Alzheimer's disease: the cost of care per patient. *Br J Health Care Manage* **4**, 332–7.

Jönsson L, Lindgren P, Wimo A, Jönsson B, Winblad B (1999a). Costs of Mini Mental State Examination – related cognitive impairment. *Pharmacoeconomics* **16**, 409–16.

Jönsson L, Lindgren P, Wimo A, Jönsson B, Winblad B (1999b). The cost-effectiveness of Donepezil therapy in Swedish patients with Alzheimer's disease: a Markov model. *Clin Ther* **21**, 1320–40.

Kavanagh S, Schneider J, Knapp M, Beecham J, Netten A (1993). Elderly people with cognitive impairment: costing possible changes in the balance of care. *Health Social Care* **1**, 69–80.

Kavanagh S and Knapp M (1999) Cognitive disability and direct costs for elderly people. *Br J Psychiatry* **174**, 539–46.

Manca A, Davies L (1999). An economic analysis of the management of Alzheimer's disease in the UK. *J Br Menopausal Soc* **5**, 167–73.

Neumann PJ, Hermann RG, Kuntz KM, et al (1999). The cost-effectiveness of Donepezil in the treatment of mild or moderate Alzheimer's disease. *Neurology* **52**, 1138–45.

[NICE] National Institute for Clinical Effectiveness (2001). *Guidance on the Use of Donepezil, Rivastigmine and Galantamine for the Treatment of Alzheimer's Disease.* Technology Assessment Guidance No. 19. London: NICE.

O'Brien BJ, Goeree R, Hux M, et al (1999). Economic evaluation of Donepezil for the treatment of Alzheimer's disease in Canada. *J Am Geriatr Soc* **47**, 570–8.

[OECD] Organization for Economic Cooperation and Development (1999). *OECD Health Data/ECO-Santé-OECD* [Data File]. Paris: OECD.

Rogers SL, Friedhoff LT (1996). The efficacy and safety of Donepezil in patients with Alzheimer's disease: results of a US multicentre, randomised, double-blind, placebo-controlled trial. *Dementia* **7**, 293–303.

Souêtre EJ, Thwaites RM, Yeardley HL (1999). Economic impact of Alzheimer's disease in the United Kingdom. Cost of care and disease severity for non-institutionalised patients with Alzheimer's disease. *Br J Psychiatry* **174**, 51–5.

Stewart A, et al (1998). Pharmacotherapy for people with Alzheimer's disease: a Markov-cycle evaluation of five years' therapy using donepezil. *Int J Geriatr Psychiatry* **13**, 445–53.

Evidence and practice

Robert Kerwin

7

Earlier chapters in this book have discussed in some detail the often conflicting clinical evidence relating to the economic consequences of using psychotropic medication in major mental illnesses. However, despite the large number of evaluations undertaken, few firm conclusions have been drawn. Without the benefit of irrefutable evidence, some might say that we should conclude nothing and base practice decisions only on the more cogent evidence available from standard clinical trials. A more realistic approach is perhaps to take into account in practice the broad outcomes of studies so far conducted while recognizing the shortfalls of the currently available data.

Schizophrenia

The advent of novel atypical antipsychotic drugs has sharpened the debate in the UK about the cost burden of schizophrenia to the National Health Service (NHS) and the relative cost-effectiveness of these drugs. Schizophrenia has a prevalence of about 0.5% and a lifetime risk of 1%. Because the disease affects adolescents and has a lifetime course associated with a high degree of hospital and social dependence it represents the second most burdensome condition after mental impairment to the NHS and social security budgets. This has been estimated at £2138 per case per year, or £396 million in direct costs (UK£, 1994 values). These direct costs represent around 2.8% of the total UK health-care budget (Knapp, 1977). This figure rises to about £1.7 billion if indirect and social costs are also taken into account (Davies and Drummond, 1994). If one looks at in-patient expenditure it is estimated that schizophrenia consumes about 5.4% of this amount. It is also apparent that over 90% of these costs are accounted for by about 50% of patients (Prudo and Bluhm, 1987; Davies and Drummond, 1994), in particular those with severe drug-refractory or intolerant illnesses. About 30% of patients are resistant to treatment (Meltzer, 1995) and a further 30% of patients are rapid relapsers within the first year of treatment (Kane et al, 1988). These figures do not include the wider costs to society such as carer burden and unemployment.

Although atypical antipsychotic agents may cost several times as much as traditional antipsychotics, drug costs in schizophrenia account for only 1–4% of the total treatment cost (Knapp, 1997). The argument then is that a small increase in drug costs—say to 10% of total cost—may result in disproportionate savings in the highly expensive direct hospital costs, if clinical trial data are translated into practical benefits. Other major costs of schizophrenia include the overall high rates of mortality and morbidity, as well as the high risk of suicide (Allebeck, 1989). Certainly, clozapine (and almost certainly other antipsychotic drugs) is associated with a lower overall risk for suicide, and the overall mortality and morbidity is also reduced (Munro et al, 1999).

If atypical antipsychotic drugs were used in all eligible patients in the UK, the prescription costs would rise by £54 million—still only a tenth or less of the total direct hospital costs. The question then arises whether this could be offset by reductions in direct costs in the face of increased indirect costs (e.g. accommodation), and whether such cost reductions could be realized in an overstretched NHS setting. Model-based analyses have demonstrated substantial potential savings for the use of clozapine (Davies and Drummond, 1994; Matheson et al, 1994). However, there are few cost-effectiveness studies in natural settings to determine if these predictions can be realized. Perhaps more importantly, it is not clear that savings in bed use would be realized in practice: it is quite possible that beds made available because of the use of clozapine will be filled by other patients requiring treatment, thereby potentially increasing costs.

Drugs available—the clinical benefit

Clozapine

Clozapine is the archetype of the atypical drugs; it was developed in the 1960s but was withdrawn from use in 1974 following reports of fatal agranulocytosis (Kerwin, 1996). Original studies comparing clozapine with a variety of typical antipsychotic drugs showed it to be either equivalent or superior in efficacy. In all cases clozapine was better tolerated (Naber et al, 2000). The best-known trial for clozapine in treatment-resistant patients was the Kane trial of 1988 where clozapine was compared with chlorpromazine in extremely resistant patients. One in three patients obtained benefit from clozapine compared with none in the chlorpromazine arm (Kane et al, 1988). Smaller studies before and since unequivocally showed benefit in treatment-resistant patients (Buchanan, 1995; Wagstaff et al, 1995). The majority of such studies show benefit for positive and negative symptoms. The Cochrane collaboration broadly concurs with this viewpoint on clozapine (Wahlbeck et al, 1999).

The drug was subsequently reintroduced for treatment-resistant or treatment-intolerant patients in the UK and USA in 1990. The drug is completely free of extrapyramidal side effects but has to be monitored for the development of neutropenia and agranulocytosis. Other problems include sialorrhoea, sedation, reduction in seizure threshold, sinus tachycardia and hepatitis. No other atypical agent has yet been shown to be comparably useful in treatment-resistant schizophrenia (e.g. Conley et al, 1998).

Risperidone

Risperidone is a benzisoxazole developed as a combined D2/5-HT$_2$ receptor blocker but with actions at a variety of other receptors (Megens et al, 1991). A range of clinical trials have shown risperidone to be effective in comparison with placebo or haloperidol. Initial studies used doses of up to 20 mg; improvement was seen in both positive and negative symptoms, while extrapyramidal side effects were seen at higher doses only (e.g. Marder and Meibach, 1994; Chouinard et al, 1993). More recently there has been interest in reducing the dose of risperidone used in clinical practice. The original trials showed the optimal dose to be about 6 mg, and 'head-to-head' studies have suggested optimal mean doses of about 7 mg (Tran et al, 1997). There is important information regarding the use of risperidone in first-episode patients, in whom it seems to be effective and free from side effects at doses of around 4–5 mg (Kopala et al, 1996). Numerous studies on risperidone in treatment-resistant patients show occasional effects but the magnitude is not as great as with clozapine. Indeed, one study showed that people who fail to improve with risperidone respond significantly to clozapine (Jeste et al, 1996; Ganguli and Brar, 1998).

Olanzapine

Olanzapine is a thienobenzodiazepine, which is chemically and pharmacologically similar to clozapine (Bymaster et al, 1996). The size and number of pivotal trials for olanzapine is impressive, although some of them have been criticized for using large doses of olanzapine (Beasley et al, 1996a, b; Tollefson et al, 1997). Again, improvements are seen in both positive and negative symptoms. The effect on negative symptoms may be particularly impressive as path analysis showed this to act on the primary deficit state rather than on secondary negative symptoms (Tollefson and Sanger, 1997). There are also good data on the long-term effects of olanzapine, with lower long-term relapse rates than haloperidol (Tran et al, 1998). An impressive study by Conley et al (1998) which copied the methodology of Kane et al (1988) failed to show any effect of olanzapine in treatment-resistant patients. Many of these patients subsequently responded to clozapine.

Quetiapine

Quetiapine is another of the $D2/5\text{-}HT_2$ blocking agents, with a multireceptor profile similar to clozapine but of generally lower overall potency (Saller and Salama, 1993). It is remarkable for its placebo-level side effect profile, and in this respect is more like clozapine than all the other atypical agents (Arvanitis and Miller, 1997). In addition, quetiapine has no effect on serum prolactin levels (Casey, 1996). There have been a number of controlled trials showing efficacy in comparison with placebo and haloperidol. The drug has a broad dose range but efficacy in most instances may not be apparent until doses of 400 mg have been reached. An unusually large number of participants drop out because of lack of drug efficacy in some of the major trials (Arvanitis and Miller, 1997).

Principally because of its efficacy/tolerability ratio, prescriptions for quetiapine are growing faster than for any other atypical antipsychotic drug at present (personal communication, Astra Zeneca).

Amisulpride

Amisulpride is a substituted benzamide, which acts as a highly selective blocker of D2 and D3 receptors (Kerwin, 2000). As with all the other drugs, it can easily be demonstrated to be effective compared with placebo and haloperidol, with a lower extrapyramidal symptom profile (Moller et al, 1995). The strength of amisulpride lies in the quality of the evidence to show that it is effective against primary negative symptoms and affective symptoms. Two studies have shown convincing superiority for negative symptoms compared with haloperidol, and there is evidence of an antidepressant effect superior not only to haloperidol but also to risperidone (Azorin, 2000).

There is evidence that amisulpride might also be useful in clozapine-resistant patients as an adjunct (Kerwin, Mathiassen and Munro, personal communication).

Cost-effectiveness of atypical antipsychotic drugs

Large numbers of cost-effectiveness studies have been performed for clozapine, presumably because this is the drug of choice in the most costly group of difficult-to-treat patients. Nearly all studies show a net saving for the use of clozapine exclusively because of the reduction in in-patient costs. Often these savings are not realized until after a year or more of treatment (Reid et al, 1994; Revicki et al, 1990). It seems that savings may be incremental for each year of treatment with clozapine (Mitchell and Munro, unpublished). In a clinic-based study comparing the 3 years prior to commencing clozapine to the period following establishment of clozapine treatment, the improvement in clinical ratings led to an average net saving per patient of £3768 per annum (Aitchison and Kerwin, 1997). This was mainly through reduction in in-patient costs despite a small accompanying increase in community costs. It remains to be seen if this theoretical effect can be realized in complex organizations with multiple cost pressures, oversubscribed beds and long waiting lists.

Pharmacoeconomic studies of other drugs are fewer and, as with clozapine, rely on less robust methods. Risperidone is probably associated with lower costs. A Swedish study applying UK costs to patient outcomes showed a reduction in mean direct costs of about £7500 per patient per year (Guest et al, 1996). Other studies, however, show risperidone to be cost-neutral (Revicki, 1999). There are fewer studies of olanzapine (although there are many publications), and taken together they suggest the drug is at least cost-neutral with respect to immediate costs (Fichner et al, 1998; Hamilton et al, 1999).

The high costs of schizophrenia have led to great economic interest in treatments both old and new. The biggest barrier to the prescribing of new drugs is probably concerns about safety and compliance, but cost is also a major factor (Kerwin, 1996). However, Knapp (1998) has noted that there is a need to know if additional treatment costs have a 'downstream' pay-off in system-wide cost-effectiveness. This is almost certainly the case for clozapine, but it is less clear for other drugs. Knapp (1998) argues that cost-effectiveness studies need to be part of the initial evaluative process rather than an afterthought. In this respect very new drugs may have an advantage as these calculations can be built into the current registration studies. However, it is my view that taking the evidence in the round for effectiveness, tolerability and cost-effectiveness, atypical antipsychotic agents are the drugs of first choice in schizophrenia.

Depression and bipolar disorder

The evidence base for clinical decisions based on cost-effectiveness for the affective disorders is less clear than for schizophrenia. In bipolar disorder the primary effectiveness of the mainstay treatments, lithium and anticonvulsant pharmacotherapy, is undergoing considerable revision (Bowden et al, 2000). Until this is clarified, cost-effectiveness studies are probably premature. Nevertheless the cost burden in bipolar disorder is qualitatively similar to that in schizophrenia, with in-patient costs being the primary burden and associated social costs in treated patients. The drug costs are even less than those for schizophrenia. In Chapter 5 John Cookson suggests there is little economic evidence to drive prescribing decisions. The in-patient burden does not seem to have altered with the introduction of lithium. The only drug-related study (Keck et al, 1996) showed an obvious difference in treatment costs only when lithium was compared with sodium valproate. Since these are both cheap drugs this is unlikely to influence clinical decisions. The main question is what impact

the atypical antipsychotics will have on the disease. A range of atypical drugs are clearly effective in bipolar disorder, and once they are licensed the way will be paved for phase 4 studies of their economic impact.

Depression is a major economic burden across the range of all health-care provision (Simon et al, 1995). The pace of drug discovery and uptake is a little more rapid than in schizophrenia, with waves of novel drugs coming along at regular intervals: tricyclic antidepressants were followed by selective serotonin reuptake inhibitors (SSRIs), followed by SNRIs, followed by the latest generation of antidepressants. Pharmacoeconomic studies are more numerous in depression than in other areas and the decisions based on these may be more sophisticated than in other areas of psychiatry (Jonsson and Rosenbaum, 1993). Quality of life and tolerability are the most important clinical and economic drivers for treatment choice in depression as the rehabilitation potential for the disease is so much greater, with most patients engaging in normal lives (Currie et al, 1993). Thus in the 1980s most psychiatrists in the developed world turned wholesale to the use of SSRIs, and attempts to persuade clinicians to use tricyclic drugs on economic grounds have largely failed. Thus a recent meta-analysis suggesting that tricyclic antidepressants are still the leading type of drug in terms of efficacy (Barbui and Hotopf, 2001) found little favour with experienced commentators (Thompson, 2001), who stated that given the enormous economic burden of depression 'the doctor's aim should be to help every patient with depression to recover and stay well at any reasonable cost.' Current questions relate to the balance of clinical and economic benefit of the newest antidepressants such as nefazodone and reboxetine. Evidence is lacking, and prescribing decisions on these new drugs should be made on individual clinical grounds. The cost differences between these and some SSRIs is minimal, therefore individual clinical considerations rather than economic factors should dominate.

Dementia

The pharmacoeconomic arguments for treating dementia are complex. There is no doubt that Alzheimer's disease represents a huge burden, between £1 billion and £6 billion per year in the UK (Manca and Davies, 1999).

Until recently there was no effective pharmacological treatment for Alzheimer's disease. Cholinesterase inhibitors are now available, but their effects are relatively small and only a proportion of patients respond (Burns et al, 1999). How should pharmacological budgets be spent on patients at the end of their life, and who should benefit when the improvements are small? Most studies showed that donepezil gave a net

clinical improvement by delaying progression to expensive forms of treatment, but in all studies this delay did not translate into potential savings (e.g. Jonsson et al, 1999). Prescribing of these drugs should therefore be on a clinical benefit basis with cost-minimization strategies. Many health authorities have developed strict criteria, usually involving recently detected patients who are not already consuming large amounts of resources, in the hope that their consumption of resources will be decelerated by the use of the drugs. It is interesting to note that the UK National Institute for Clinical Effectiveness has approved the use of these drugs in the NHS, albeit with provisos (specialist use, etc.), on clinical and cost-effectiveness grounds.

Anxiety disorders

This topic has already been well summarized in Chapter 4 by Malcolm Lader. The anxiety disorders have generally received little attention, and treatment decisions are complicated by the heterogeneity of the different disorders, some being more biological than others. It is now clear that the cost-benefit ratio for benzodiazepines is adverse in the long term, and in any case there are good cost-effectiveness studies in generalized anxiety that show both clinical and economic superiority for psychological treatments (Gould et al, 1995).

Pharmacologically, a principal point relates to the cost-effectiveness of the newer indications for SSRIs in the less common disorders such as obsessive–compulsive disorder and social phobia. These conditions do place a disproportionate burden on health-care systems, and clinical trials of the newer indications are convincing. However, no cost-effectiveness study has yet been performed to assess this, and prescribing will continue to be based on individual clinical need.

Conclusion

Pharmacoeconomics is a nascent discipline which has not yet provided clinicians and budget managers with the level of information necessary for confident decision-making. This is particularly true in psychiatry where the dearth of acceptable, reliably measurable clinical end points makes pharmacoeconomic evaluation even more complex and open to debate. Nonetheless, the data reviewed in this book, when placed alongside clinical data, do provide a framework for decision-making which is better informed and more realistic than any exclusively clinical assessment could be. Economic evaluations in all major mental illnesses, while some way from conclusive, are certainly providing valuable guidance to decision-makers both at policy level and in the clinic.

References

Aitchison KJ, Kerwin RW (1997). Cost effectiveness of clozapine. A UK based clinic study. *Br J Psychiatry* **171**, 125–30.

Allebeck P (1989). Schizophrenia: A life shortening disease. *Schizophr Bull* **15**, 81–9.

Arvanitis LA, Miller BG (1997). Multiple fixed doses of seroquel (quetiapine) in patients with acute exacerbations of schizophrenia. A comparison with haloperidol and placebo. The seroquel trial 13 study group. *Biol Psychiatry* **42**, 233–46.

Azorin JM (2000). Acute phase of schizophrenia. Impact of atypical antipsychotics. *Int Clin Psychopharmacol* **15** (suppl. 4), 11–14.

Barbui C, Hotopf M (2001). Amitriptyline v. the rest: still leading the world after 40 years of randomised controlled trials. *Br J Psychiatry* **178**, 129–44.

Beasley C, Sanger T, Satterlee W, et al (1996a). Olanzapine vs placebo: results of a double blind fixed dose olanzapine trial. *Psychopharmacology* **124**, 159–67.

Beasley CM, Tollefson G, Tran P, et al (1996b). Olanzapine vs placebo and haloperidol. Acute phase results of the North American double blind olanzapine trial. *Neuropsychopharmacology* **14**, 111–23.

Bowden CL, Calabrese JR, McElroy SL, et al (2000). A randomised placebo controlled 12 month trial of divalproex and lithium in treatment of outpatients with bipolar 1 disorder. *Arch Gen Psychiatry* **57**, 481–9.

Buchanan RW (1995). Clozapine: efficacy and safety. *Schizophr Bull* **21**, 579–91.

Burns A, Russell E, Page S (1999). New drugs for Alzheimers disease. *Br J Psychiatry* **174**, 476–9.

Bymaster F, Calligaro DO, Falcone JF, et al (1996). Radioreceptor binding profile of the atypical antipsychotic olanzapine. *Neuropsychopharmacology* 14, 87–96.

Casey DE (1996). Seroquel (quetiapine). Preclinical and clinical findings of a new atypical antipsychotic. *Expert Opin Invest Drugs* 5, 939–57.

Chouinard G, Jones B, Remington G, et al (1993). A Canadian multicentre placebo controlled study of fixed doses of risperidone and haloperidol in the treatment of chronic schizophrenic inpatients. *J Clin Psychopharmacol* 13, 25–40.

Conley RR, Tamminga CA, Bartko JJ, et al (1998). Olanzapine compared with chlorpromazine in treatment resistant schizophrenia. *Am J Psychiatry* 155, 914–20.

Currie DJ, Fairweather DB, Hindmarch I (1993). Social aspects of treating depression. In: Jonsson B, Rosenbaum J, eds, *The Health Economics of Depression.* New York: Wiley, 129–40.

Davies LM, Drummond MF (1994). Economics and schizophrenia. The real cost. *Br J Psychiatry* 165 (suppl. 25), 18–21.

Fichner CG, Hanrahan P, Luchins DJ (1998). Pharmacoeconomic studies of atypical antipsychotics. *Psychiatr Ann* 28, 381–96.

Ganguli R, Brar JS (1998). The effects of risperidone and olanzapine on the indications for clozapine. *Psychopharmacol Bull* 34, 83–7.

Gould RA, Otto MW, Pollack MH (1995). A meta analysis of treatment outcome for panic disorder. *Clin Psychol Rev* 15, 819–44.

Guest JF, Hart WM, Cookson RF, et al (1996). Pharmacoeconomic evaluation of long term treatment with risperidone for patients with chronic schizophrenia. *Br J Med Econ* 10, 59–67.

Jeste DV, Klausner M, Brecher M, et al (1996). A clinical evaluation of risperidone in the treatment of schizophrenia: a ten week open label multicentre trial. *Psychopharmacology* 131, 239–47.

Jonsson B, Rosenbaum J eds (1993). *The Health Economics of Depression.* New York: Wiley.

Jonsson L, Lindgren P, Wimo A, et al (1999). The cost effectiveness of donepezil therapy in Swedish patients with Alzheimers disease. *Clin Ther* 21, 1320–40.

Hamilton SH, Revicki DA, Edgell ET, et al (1999). Clinical and economic outcomes of olanzapine compared with haloperidol for schizophrenia: results from a randomised clinical trial. *Pharmacoeconomics* 15, 469–80.

Kane J, Honigfeld G, Singer J, et al (1988). Clozapine for the treatment resistant schizophrenic. A double blind comparison with chlorpromazine. *Arch Gen Psychiatry* 33, 766–71.

Keck PE, McElroy SL, Bennett JA (1996). Health economic implications of the onset of action of antimanic agents. *J Clin Psychiatry* 57 (suppl. 13), 13–18.

Kerwin RW (1996). An essay on the new antipsychotics. *Psychiatr Bull* 20, 23–9.

Kerwin RW (2000). Amisulpride: from pharmacological profiles to clinical outcome. *Int Clin Psychopharmacol* 15 (suppl. 4), 1–4.

Knapp MRJ (1997). Costs of schizophrenia. *Br J Psychiatry* 171, 509–18.

Knapp MRJ (1998). Measuring the economic benefit of treatment with atypical antipsychotics. *Eur Psychiatry* 13 (suppl. 1), 37–45s.

Kopala LC, Fredrikson D, Good KP, Honer WG (1996). Symptoms in neuroleptic naïve first episode schizophrenia: response to risperidone. *Biol Psychiatry* **39**, 296–8.

Manca A, Davies L (1999). An economic analysis of the management of Alzheimers disease in the UK. *J Br Menopausal Soc* **5**, 167–73.

Marder S, Meibach RC (1994). Risperidone in the treatment of schizophrenia. *Am J Psychiatry* **151**, 825–35.

Matheson LA, Cook HM, McKenna P, et al (1994). Value for money for patients with schizophrenia. *Br J Med Econ* 7, 25–34.

Megens AAHP, Awouters FHI, Schotte A, et al (1991). A survey on the pharmacodynamics of the new antipsychotic risperidone. *Psychopharmacology* **114**, 9–23.

Meltzer H (1995). The concept of atypical antipsychotics. In: Jaden Boer, Westenberg HGM, van Praag HM, eds, *Advances in the Neurobiology of Schizophrenia*, vol. 1. Chichester: Wiley, 265–73.

Moller HJ, Muller H, Borison RL, et al (1995). A path analytical approach to differentiate between direct and indirect drug effects on negative symptoms in schizophrenic patients: a re-evaluation of the North American Risperidone study. *Eur Arch Psychiatry Clin Neurol* 245, 45–9.

Munro J, O'Sullivan D, Andrews C, et al (1999). Active monitoring of 12760 clozapine recipients in the UK and Ireland. *Br J Psychiatry* **175**, 576–80.

Naber D, Haasen C, Perro C (2000). Clozapine. The first atypical antipsychotic. In: Ellenbrook BA, Cools AR, eds, *Atypical Antipsychotics*. Basel: Birkhauser, 145–62.

Prudo R, Bluhm HM (1987). Five year outcome and prognosis in schizophrenia. *Br J Psychiatry* **150**, 345–54.

Reid WH, Mason M, Topral M (1994). Savings in hospital bed days related to treatment with clozapine. *Hosp Community Psychiatry* **45**, 261–4.

Revicki DA (1999). Pharmacoeconomic studies of atypical antipsychotic drugs for the treatment of schizophrenia. *Schizophr Res* **35** (suppl.), s101–9.

Revicki DA, Luce BR, Wechsler JM, et al (1990). Cost effectiveness of clozapine for treatment resistant schizophrenic patients. *Hosp Community Psychiatry* **41**, 850–69.

Saller CF, Salama AI (1993). Seroquel: biochemical profile of a potential atypical antipsychotic. *Psychopharmacology* **112**, 285–8.

Simon G, Wagner E, Von Korff M (1995). Cost effectiveness comparisons using real world randomised trials: the case of new antidepressant drugs. *J Clin Epidemiol* **48**, 363–73.

Thompson C (2001). Amitriptyline: still efficacious, but at what cost? *Br J Psychiatry* **178**, 99–100.

Tollefson GD, Sanger TM (1997). Negative symptoms: a path analytic approach to a double blind, placebo controlled clinical trial with olanzapine. *Am J Psychiatry* **154**, 466–74.

Tollefson GD, Beasley CM, Tran PV, et al (1997). Olanzapine vs haloperidol in the treatment of schizophrenia and schizoaffective and schizophreniform disorders. Results of an international collaborative trial. *Am J Psychiatry* **154**, 457–65.

Tran PV, Hamilton SH, Kuntz AJ, et al (1997). Double blind comparison of olanzapine vs risperidone in the treatment of schizophrenia and other psychotic disorders. *J Clin Psychopharmacol* **17**, 407–18.

Tran PV, Dellva MA, Tollefson GD, et al (1998). Oral olanzapine vs oral haloperidol in the maintenance treatment of schizophrenia. *Br J Psychiatry* **172**, 499–505.

Wagstaff AJ, Bryson HM (1995). Clozapine—a review of its pharmacological properties and therapeutic use in patients with schizophrenia who are unresponsive to or intolerant of classical antipsychotic agents. *CNS Drugs* **4**, 370–400.

Wahlbeck K, Cheine M, Essali A, Adams C (1999). Evidence of clozapine's effectiveness in schizophrenia: a systematic review and meta-analysis of randomised trials. *Am J Psychiatry* **156**, 990–9.

Index